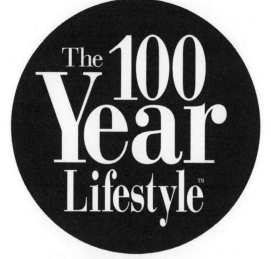

WORKOUT

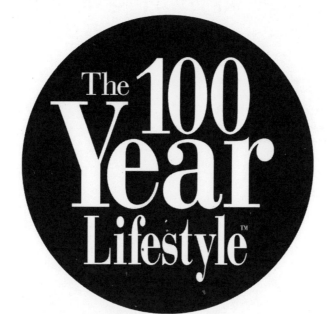

WORKOUT

The High Energy Fitness Program for Living at Your Peak Throughout Your Lifetime

ERIC PLASKER, DC,

Internationally Acclaimed Wellness Expert

life

Guilford, Connecticut
An imprint of Globe Pequot Press

life

GPP Life is an imprint of Globe Pequot Press.

Photos by Alan Lemberger
Text designed by Sheryl P. Kober
Layout by Melissa Evarts

Library of Congress Cataloging-in-Publication Data is available on file.

ISBN 978-0-7627-5273-7

Printed in the United States of America

10 9 8 7 6 5 4 3 2 1

I dedicate this book to all the doctors of chiropractic, medical doctors, personal trainers, and other health and fitness professionals around the world who see beyond politics and who work hard to change peoples lives every day for the better. May you continue to lead our society to better health.

In memory of Dr. Joseph Flesia

I think of you every day. Your passion, vision, and strategies inspire my work and fuel my commitment to solving the predicament of the species.

CONTENTS

INTRODUCTION

I remember the first time I heard about the possibility of people living beyond the age of 100. I was at a seminar listening to Dr. Joseph Flesia speak about a group of people on the other side of the world in the mountains of northern Pakistan. They were called the Hunzas and they lived "well" to well over 100 years old—disease free. Back in the seventies, as part of a series of reports on living longer, *National Geographic* wrote about them, marveling at the longevity this group of people seemed to possess genetically.

What were their secrets? Everyone wanted to know. The fact that they lived on the other side of the planet in a small village in the mountains, made the group very intriguing to western culture. Could the answers lie solely in their genes? Or, did lifestyle play a role in their life span and if so how much of a role?

While studying longevity, I learned that research by the MacArthur Foundation found that quality of life and longevity is 30 percent genetics and 70 percent lifestyle. The Hunzas were blessed with excellent genes for longevity, but they also made self-care a priority through healthy eating, physical activity, and a strong social circle of family and community. And they maintained a sense of balance between work and the other elements of their lives. Without calling it such, they had lived The 100 Year Lifestyle described in my first book.

Their biggest secret to their longevity success: They were fit! They lived an active healthy lifestyle, yet they were not drug takers or gym rats. They weren't ripped with every muscle striation popping through their skin. They worked in the mountains or fields, lived off the land, spent only a few hours sitting on their bottoms, and lived relatively stress-free lives.

This isn't the way our modern culture lives. In fact, the western world spends an extraordinary amount of time sitting. According to the President's Council on Physical Fitness and Sports, the United States will spend $1.5 trillion over the next ten years treating conditions that result from a sedentary lifestyle. We have become an obese nation.

According to the December 1, 2008, issue of *Time*, which covered the sorry state of American health, only 33 percent of adults are at their ideal weight. That means that 67 percent of adults are overweight. Nearly 20 percent of kids are obese, and a staggering 32 percent of American kids are overweight, making them more prone to heart disease and diabetes among other preventable diseases.

THE 100 YEAR LIFESTYLE

When I wrote *The 100 Year Lifestyle*, it was intended to be much more than a book. It was intended to define a brand new health care model for a world of extended life spans. I am excited to see this happening on a grass roots level around the globe.

My chiropractic practice exposed me to the importance of lifestyle and healthy aging. Patients would come in feeling the excruciating pain of arthritis, and through their chiropractic care and lifestyle changes they would feel better, younger, and healthier, even though their age was the same. I would see people with "genetic" conditions, such as heart disease and cancer, change their lifestyle and become healthy again, even though their genes were the same. One child who was diagnosed with a genetic condition adopted the lifestyle changes we discuss in *The 100 Year Lifestyle* and *The 100 Year Lifestyle Workout,* and his entire demeanor changed. While he still had the genetic condition, the lifestyle changes that he and his family made together improved their health and quality of life dramatically. Through The 100 Year Lifestyle, they were able to maximize the expression of their genes.

I have seen athletes improve their strength, times, and stamina through lifestyle changes, setting personal records that they only dreamed of. I have seen people permanently remove excess weight, lower their cholesterol naturally, and see their own bodies heal from nearly every type of health problem. I have cared for patients who have outlived their parents and their grandparents, some of them suffering in their longevity while others, living The 100 Year Lifestyle, made the most of their extended lives. I have also seen numerous patients who would blame their genes for conditions like diabetes, heart disease, and herniated discs to name a few, who blamed their parents for these conditions, while it was really an unhealthy lifestyle that they inherited.

A lifestyle of unhealthy eating, stress, excessive sitting, or improper lifting can take its toll on even the best genetic specimen. We've all heard the expression that it's not the cards you've been dealt but how you play them that matters most. You can't control the genes you have inherited, but you can choose how you play them through the lifestyle that you choose to live.

Now, more than ever, it's time for us to fully embrace The 100 Year Lifestyle. After all, nobody wants to get to 100, or even sixty, seventy, or eighty for that matter, crippled, broke, or alone. Fitness centers, doctors of chiropractors, medical doctors, personal trainers, relationship counselors, massage therapists, and many other types of health and wellness professionals are using my first book to educate their patients and clients about their health, quality of life, and longevity. Even financial planners are using the book to stress to their clients the importance of adjusting their financial plan for 100 years and beyond.

Many fitness centers and personal training studios are making The 100 Year Lifestyle a part of their corporate culture. Since the Lifestyle Fitness Plan of Getting Your ESS in Shape is one of the most talked-about sections of the original 100 Year Lifestyle book, I decided to expand on it and write *The 100 Year Lifestyle Workout.* I hope this edition will inspire you to add to the changes you've already made from the first book, or inspire those of you reading for the first time to make a change toward the quality of life and longevity you deserve. It's that longevity and attention to fitness and health that could make us all a generation of *American* Hunzas.

THE 100 YEAR LIFESTYLE WORKOUT

What's unique about *The 100 Year Lifestyle Workout?* This lifestyle, nutrition, and fitness program is designed to get you in the best shape of your life regardless of your age and keep you that way for a lifetime. It will break you through health and fitness plateaus and get you off the weight gain/weight loss roller coaster. It will give you the mindset and focus to make fitness a part of your lifestyle and to enjoy it, rather than have it feel like a burden. You will look great, and you will love it! The workout is for everyone, especially Baby Boomers who aren't as young as you used to be, but who want to act and feel like you are. You want to get in or stay in shape. While many of you may have old injuries, *The 100 Year Lifestyle Workout* will provide you with the ability to adapt your workouts to your injuries and your age. It will also help lay the groundwork for an active lifestyle into your later years.

Get Your ESS in Shape—Unique and Vital to Healthy Aging

The ESS concept is the framework for *The 100 Year Lifestyle Workout.* It involves the three elements that must be in shape to ensure quality of life as people age, namely your Endurance, Strength, and Structure. Endurance relates to good cardiovascular exercise, important for a healthy heart. Strength covers strength training, a component of being able to stay healthy, active, and mobile as you age, and Structure deals with posture, flexibility, a healthy muscular system, and a healthy spine and nervous system. The balance between the three, the ESS, ensures

good health, mobility, and activity as you age. An unhealthy heart, weak muscles and bones, or a deteriorated spine can all severely limit your quality of life today and certainly as you age. Balancing all three of these components in your workouts and your life is vital.

With the instability and uncertainty of our financial and health care systems, your personal fitness is more important than ever, and it is your responsibility. Baby Boomers have a legitimate concern about the stability of Social Security and Medicare and The 100 Year Lifestyle Workout is designed with this in mind. It provides a foundation that will allow you to adapt your workout as you age and adapt to injuries or illnesses if they arise. *The 100 Year Lifestyle Workout* provides you with the knowledge, tools, and structure you need to implement The 100 Year Lifestyle on a whole new level and make the most of your innate, genetic potential.

Baby Boomers are also seeing the declining health and function of their aging parents and grandparents. They are having heart problems, strength issues as they struggle to get out of a chair, and spinal health issues as they become hunched over. This is causing Boomers to make their health and fitness a priority and take matters into their own hands.

It doesn't matter what your starting point is. Get ready to get your ESS in the best shape of your life and enjoy the health, vitality, and energy that comes with living your ideal 100 Year Lifestyle.

See you there!

Dr. Eric Plasker

CHAPTER ONE:

Love Your Age. Adjust Your Lifestyle.

Welcome to *The 100 Year Lifestyle Workout.* Whether you are brand new to The 100 Year Lifestyle or you have been one of our loyal, enthusiastic followers, I want you to think about that incredibly provocative question that we asked you at the beginning of the first book. "If you knew you would live to be 100, how would you change your life?"

If you are like most people, you will examine your health, your relationships, your vitality, your energy, the way you earn income, the social circles that you function in, as well as the lifestyle that you want to live during your extended life span. Lots of things may filter through your mind. Maybe you need to change your job. Maybe you need to improve the quality of your relationships, speak up for yourself, or take on a new career. And maybe, just maybe, you recognize that it's time to get your ESS in shape—your Endurance, Strength, and Structure.

Well today, with The 100 Year Lifestyle Workout, it's time for you to decide. I want you to decide once and for all that you are going to make fitness and keeping your ESS in shape a part of your lifestyle from this point forward.

How old are you? I know this is a politically incorrect question, but regardless of the number, it's time to love your age. It's yours. Adjust your lifestyle so that you make the best of every day and ensure that your best years are yet to come.

The fitness revolution is booming and you probably know that you need to be exercising. You are fully aware that fitness should be a part of your lifestyle. Are you doing what you know? Are you living what you know? Regardless of your age and current health condition this book will take you on a journey to get you in the best shape of your life. You will love it. And if you don't love it or are concerned that you won't love it, you will learn to love it because you will begin to think differently and experience a greater quality of life, which is a very lovable concept. And this is certainly much better than the alternative.

Over the past two years, I have traveled the world and seen people during every stage of their life change their life and become more fit and healthy than ever. Fitness is a decision. Living The 100 Year Lifestyle is a decision. On the other hand, living a forty, fifty, or sixty year lifestyle or living a lifestyle of poor quality regardless of your age may not have been a decision for you. Somehow, some way maybe you set out on a path that was destructive to your mind and your body. Maybe you became complacent and somehow found yourself a couch potato, and you unconsciously became a hidden number in the epidemic of obesity that is plaguing our nation. If this happened to you

ESS Story: Jack LaLanne

For nearly my entire seventy-year career, my mission has been to help people help themselves to feel better, look better, and live longer. I have been blessed to be able to motivate millions of people through my health clubs, television shows, radio shows, and the Stay Fit Seniors exercise program. In essence, I have been telling the world to live The 100 Year Lifestyle. And while I have received numerous honors in my lifetime including receiving a star on the Hollywood Walk of Fame and the Arnold Classic Lifetime Achievement Award, nothing makes me happier than seeing people change their life for the better.

I wasn't always healthy. As a child I was addicted to sugar and junk food and my unhealthy lifestyle wreaked havoc on my life. It affected my schoolwork, my relationships with my family, teachers, and friends, and today I might have been prescribed a lifetime of hyperactivity drugs. Instead, at the age of fifteen, I was fortunate enough to hear a gentleman by the name of Paul Bragg speak about health and it had a positive impact on my life, changing me forever. I became motivated to learn as much about health, fitness, quality of life, and

longevity as I possibly could. I committed myself to "getting my ESS in shape" through weightlifting and good nutrition, which was unheard of in the 1930s. I went to chiropractic college to learn the importance of having a healthy spine and nervous system, where I studied *Gray's Anatomy* to learn about the nerves, muscles, and organ systems. I applied these principles to not only help myself but to also help people in my community. The principles that I learned, studied, and chose to live are the principles that Dr. Plasker talks about in *The 100 Year Lifestyle* that every individual should live regardless of their age.

The ESS principles of Endurance, Strength, and Structure in *The 100 Year Lifestyle Workout* are very similar to the core principles that I used to open my first health club in 1936. They are similar principles to the ones that I used in all of the fitness firsts that I have been able to accomplish in my lifetime, including opening the first modern day health spa, being the first to have a nationally syndicated exercise show on television, being the first to have athletes, women, and the elderly work out with weights, and, yes, I was also the first to put a health food bar in a gym, come up with weight loss and healthy meal replacement drinks, and many other firsts that are just too numerous to name. All of these with a mission of helping people look and feel their best for a long healthy life.

It breaks my heart that we have an obesity epidemic in the United States of America and in industrialized communities worldwide. This is not necessary and I believe that if people understood their own human potential then they would adopt the principles in this book. I strongly believe in every individual's human potential and that people should pursue their own potential throughout their lives. The 100 Year Lifestyle is a great tool to help you do that.

My amazing feats of strength and endurance, such as swimming the length of the Golden Gate Bridge underwater with 140 pounds of equipment on my back, swimming handcuffed and shackled pulling a 1,000-pound boat from Alcatraz to Fisherman's Wharf, and setting the world record of 1,033 situps in 23 minutes and 53 seconds were not designed to be just about me. I wanted to show people what was possible if they took care of their bodies and

their minds and if they believed and nurtured their own potential. Don't settle for anything less than this for yourself, especially your quality of life as you age.

You can change your life through this book and through these principles no matter what your age, if you are willing to make the commitment and change your lifestyle. Even now, healthy at age ninety-four, my wife Elaine and I remain committed to my mission. Through Stay Fit Seniors, the health and fitness program that is attaching to doctors' offices and municipalities around the country, the eighty million seniors will have a place where they can get and keep their ESS in shape and make the rest of their life the best of their life. It is never too late to live these principles and to apply the principles of The 100 Year Lifestyle.

Anything is possible and you can make it happen. Don't waste another minute, hour, day, month, or year. And as Dr. Plasker would say, enjoy a sensational century! See you there!

Jack LaLanne
www.jacklalanne.com
www.stayfitseniors.com

it's time to get your life back. It's time to regain consciousness and make a decision.

You will love the information and the fitness plan that you are about to embrace. Maybe you are one of those people who wants to maximize your innate potential and the expression of your genes so you can get the most out of your life, your mind, and your body. Either way, you will be excited about this journey that we are about to embark on together.

Get yourself a partner or two or three to embrace this journey with you. Doing The 100 Year Lifestyle Workout program with your family, your friends, and even your coworkers will help you build a surround sound system of support filled with the constant positive energy and vitality that will sustain you on the days when things get tough and your mind is somehow brought back into the gutter. Stick with me and stick with this program and get excited to get your ESS in the best shape of your life.

Is your story different than Jack LaLanne's? Mine sure is. I was fit as a kid, participating in sports and bodybuilding, and very active on every level. When I went to chiropractic college, I remained fit and healthy and was excited about the opportunity to help people live better quality lives through my training as a doctor of chiropractic and wellness specialist. In 1991, ten months after my oldest child was born, he had an accident that left him paralyzed. We were told by the greatest medical experts in Atlanta that he would never walk, never talk, and never use his arm. Thanks to my training as a chiropractor and a wellness expert, combined with my wife Lisa's determined spirit and relentless efforts, and Jacob's innate healing abilities, he is now nineteen years old and a healthy, highly functional, college student at the University of Georgia. His story has inspired people around the globe.

During his healing and for a decade afterwards, my focus on my own health slipped. I gained nearly forty pounds, taking care of everyone in my family but myself. On my son's thirteenth birthday, we made a video in his honor, and watching myself on the big screen that day in 2002 was the day that changed my life. I decided to begin living the message that I was preaching to all of my patients once again. Now at forty-six, I am in nearly the best shape of my life and getting better every day. Those forty pounds have been gone for five years and I feel younger and healthier than ever. Through The 100 Year Lifestyle Workout, you too can get in the best shape of your life, no matter what your age or current health condition.

DO YOU LIKE WHAT YOU SEE?

Do a "full being" survey on yourself and decide if you like what you see. Examine your body, mind, and spirit. Look down at your gut. Is it hanging over your belt or are you tight and lean? Look around your eyes. Have the stress lines taken over or are you relaxed and happy? Look at your spine. Is your posture deteriorating or are you able to stand straight effortlessly? Are your hips and shoulders level or are they unbalanced? Are you starting to develop a hunchback? Look deeper. Do you see a happy person with radiant energy or are you buried beneath a cushion of extra pounds and unconscious suffering?

If you like what you see, get ready to take your health to the next level and enjoy the best years of your life. If you don't like what you see, then stop blaming your genes. It's not their fault. It is your choices, your lifestyle's fault. Are you making the most of your genes? Are you living your genetic potential?

The 100 Year Lifestyle Workout is more than just a physical workout—way more. It is a philosophy and lifestyle model that you and your family can live to maximize the expression of your genes. It is a total lifestyle approach to getting the most out of your life, while you also give the most with your life. Now is your time to embrace your longevity and make the changes to your lifestyle that will help you make the most of your extended life span.

The 100 Year Lifestyle Defined

WHAT IT IS . . .
- Living a healthy, passionate, prosperous life, every day of your life, for 100 years and beyond
- Great relationships with multiple generations and multiple circles of people
- Lifelong learning, activity, and adventure
- Financial freedom, abundance, and independence
- The perfect balance of exploration, play time, and fun combined with meaningful work
- Maximizing your genetic capabilities and making the most of your time, energy, and talents
- Keeping your original body parts functioning at full capacity
- Stimulating your mind to keep it sharp
- Accepting challenges, embracing change, and adapting to the unexpected
- Balancing the need for immediate gratification and a secure future
- Knowing and trusting yourself
- Yours to customize

WHAT IT IS NOT . . .
- Rotting away as a human preservative in a nursing home
- Abusing your body, masking symptoms with drugs, and then continuing to abuse yourself until one organ after the other has to be removed or replaced
- All work and no play
- Abusive relationships or isolation
- Financial survival for thirty-five years and then barely squeaking by on Social Security and Medicare
- Insignificant retirement where you become a meaningless number in a long line of an outdated system
- Wearing out your body in the first fifty years and then suffering the consequences during the second fifty years
- Accumulating wealth in the first fifty years and destroying relationships along the way, leaving you nobody to share it with
- Creating wealth at the price of your health
- Denying yourself the good things in life

What 100 Year Lifestylers Are Saying

The comments I've heard from my readers since *The 100 Year Lifestyle* came out have been amazing. I hear people say things all the time like . . .

- "It's great to get my youthful spirit back."
- "I feel younger and healthier than I have in twenty years."
- "My energy level has skyrocketed."
- "I've lost so much weight."
- "I am feeling more confident in myself."
- "I am excited, rather than afraid, of getting older."
- "I have a vision for my life."
- "I am starting a new business."
- "I have reconnected with our friends."
- "I finally have balance in my life."
- "My marriage is better than ever."
- "I am a happier person."
- "I finally ended a destructive relationship."
- "I feel great."

Isn't it amazing what can happen when you embrace the possibility of living for thirty, forty, fifty, or even sixty more years?

YOU CAN DO IT, TOO!

Get ready to experience what so many people already have. If your lifestyle has taken a turn for the worse then your genetics probably followed. It's not too late to reverse the momentum. Your body has within it an innate intelligence that guides your genes to adapt to your lifestyle. In the past, your genes may have adapted to your lifestyle in what you perceive to be a negative way. If you have been eating too much, your body adapted by storing all those excess calories as fat, because it thinks you may need them during an extended hibernation stay in a cave. While this is not healthy for you in the long run, it is not the adaptation that's going to kill you, it's the poor habits.

If you have been sitting too much and you are living a sedentary lifestyle, your body adapted by padding your bottom. While certainly this is unhealthy, it is the appropriate adaptation based on the lifestyle you have been living. If you have been slouching all day, your body probably adapted by growing your spine and your muscles for stability around this unhealthy posture, and even though it is not the ideal posture for your quality of life to 100 years and beyond, it was the adaptation that was necessary for your genes to sustain you based on your choices and your lifestyle.

Fortunately your poor lifestyle choices didn't kill you yet, which is great news for you. Rather your body adapted by storing more fat, clogging your arteries, or causing minor misalignments in your spine, putting pressure on your nerves by growing crooked.

The good news is that even if you don't like the way your body adapted, it is certainly better than the alternative. Once you get started with the Workout, your genes will adapt again, to your new lifestyle. Your body will get smaller and tighter if you adjust your lifestyle. If you are willing to make the changes that support the optimum expression of your genes, you will maximize both the length and quality of your life.

You are a vital, energetic being. When you focus and harness this energy in a healthy way, your incredible innate intelligence will use this energy to fuel your sensational century. To do this, you have to be healthy. Decide to harness this energy for health. Use it to get fit, stay fit, and keep you active and healthy for a lifetime.

Set yourself free. If you have burdens that you are holding onto, they will weigh you down and show up on the scale. Burdens consume your energy. They are responsible for habits that add extra fat to your body so that you can have a little extra protection. Get ready to let go and embrace the best years of your life.

YOU CAN'T AFFORD TO GET SICK

The economy is affecting everyone. People are shopping more strategically, they are getting their financial affairs more organized, and they are cutting back on the frills in their life to hunker down. A lot of people are wondering what they should cut out, what they should cut back on, and what they should include in their budget so they can make ends meet. "I can't afford it" are common words that I hear people use as they try to make sense of the lifestyle adjustments that they need to make. What should they do with their gym membership, organic foods, exercise equipment, chiropractic care? People are wondering whether or not they can afford to continue with their healthy lifestyle.

With all the uncertainty out there in the market, there is absolutely, positively one thing that you cannot afford in our country today. You cannot afford to get sick!!!

According to a recent *Reader's Digest* article, 70 percent of those people who went into debt due to a medical condition had health insurance at the time. Of those surveyed, 49 percent said they put off or refused medical treatment for a serious condition because of money. A hip replacement costs in the neighborhood of $49,000 not including the rehabilitation, lost time off work, and lost quality of life. You should be crystal clear about the fact that in this economy, especially when you consider the probability of living an extended life span, you cannot afford to get sick, and that keeping yourself healthy is one of the most important things you can do for yourself and your family.

So, what should you do to keep yourself healthy and what should your priorities be? Your fitness should be one of your top priorities. If you've lost your job and you need to begin searching for a new place to work or a new career, you will be more confident if you are fit. You will present yourself in a more positive, healthy light. To whom might a prospective employer offer a job if they had two people with the same college degree, the same work experience, and the same qualifications? The fit and healthy person or the overweight, stressed out person? If you have been out of work, it is more important than ever to get your ESS in shape if you want your life to change. A recent *Time* magazine discussed the top ten ideas that were changing the world. Number nine on the list was mandatory health; the article stated that companies and organizations were starting to adopt policies and protocols that established an environment of health and fitness. On the job training is taking on a whole new meaning as more and more companies are making fitness in the workplace a priority. It is exciting to see many 100 Year Lifestyle providers leading the way by providing the education and information to companies who want to create a healthier culture for their employees.

START THINKING ABOUT WHAT AND HOW YOU EAT

Don't diet. Make healthy eating a part of your lifestyle. Too many people will only eat healthy when they get sick or get fat. They will starve themselves or force down healthy foods to lose weight, get in shape, or heal from their disease. Because they are, in their own mind, depriving themselves from the "treats" that they are used to eating, they suffer through their deprivation and bail out on their healthy eating plan the second their skinny jeans fit, only to repeat

this roller coaster a few months later. Many of the foods we think are treats are really tricks in disguise. Are two minutes of pleasurable taste worth weeks of low self-esteem and frustration because you don't look or feel the way that you want? Make healthy eating a part of your lifestyle. This book will give you excellent healthy eating strategies.

MAKE EXERCISE A PART OF YOUR LIFESTYLE

When you look at the top ten leading causes of death in this country, nine out of ten of them are preventable with a healthy lifestyle. Lack of exercise is on the list as a contributor to every single one of them except for unintentional injuries. It is time that you make exercise a part of your lifestyle. Make movement a part of your lifestyle.

In addition to your workouts, go for a ten-minute walk after your meals. Do a ten-minute stretch after you've been sitting for an extended period of time.

Remember the three components of exercise that you must keep in mind for a healthy workout are your ESS: Endurance, Strength, and Structure. All three of these components are essential to quality of life as you age, while also preventing unnecessary injuries or sickness. Here is a basic overview, and we will cover this in greater detail later in this book.

Good cardiovascular exercise, such as running, swimming, power walking, or a game of basketball or tennis, helps create endurance. If you have had any previous injuries, you can do low-impact endurance training on an elliptical, a bike, or a treadmill. Strength training is equally important. A stronger body is more resistant to stress. You will need your strength to ensure quality of life as you age. Structure is also important because you have to take care of your core, and you have to take care of your spine and nervous system. Americans spend nearly $90 billion looking for a solution to back-related health problems, many of which can be prevented with proper care. To ensure your quality of life as you age, you must balance all three elements of The 100 Year Lifestyle Workout.

THERE IS VALUE IN STAYING HEALTHY

Learning and living The 100 Year Lifestyle Workout is the best investment you can make in yourself. Unfortunately for our modern day culture—both here and in many industrialized nations—there's a longevity crisis. People are living longer whether they like it or not, and they haven't invested in making those extra years healthy ones. You're probably experiencing this on some level in your own life, watching your parents or grandparents age, their bodies and minds not prepared to reach eighty, ninety, or 100 years and beyond.

The number of nursing homes and assisted living centers that are popping up everywhere is astounding. There are 1.5 million people living in nursing homes in the United States. Forty-six percent of them are over the age of eighty-five. By the year 2050 an estimated sixty million people will be over the age of eighty. This last number probably includes you. The current generation of seniors, centenarians, and super-centenarians (110 years old and older) is growing. Unfortunately, these unsuspecting souls were blindsided by their longevity and not prepared for their extra years. You don't have to be. We are getting the advance notice that our parents and grandparents never received that our innate genetic potential for longevity is well beyond 100 years and that, with the right lifestyle choices and a little luck, they can be healthy and enjoyable years.

You can't believe how many times I've heard the joke from our loyal readers and followers, "hey Dr. P, I am writing the sequel, *The 101 Year Lifestyle*" or *"The 110 Year Lifestyle"* or even *"The 150 Year Lifestyle."* The reality is, if you live The 100 Year Lifestyle and make it to 100 with your health, energy, vitality, and with vision for your life, you may defy our current scientific knowledge and beliefs about what the upward limit on longevity may actually be. Remember, our current generation of centenarians outlived their life expectancy by five decades. They did it by accident. We can do it in style.

The 100 Year Lifestyle isn't about getting to 100 and then dropping dead at the finish line after a deteriorating last decade. It's really about living your best life every day of your life and making the most of your genetic potential regardless of your age. Keeping yourself fit and healthy is at the core of this lifestyle and it is essential to ensure your personal confidence and your ability to enjoy quality of life now, and as you age. It is also important for your children, grandchildren, and for some of you, your great grandchildren, who are growing up in unhealthy homes with unhealthy lifestyles. No wonder there is a concern about the current generation of kids, who may be the first generation in decades whose life expectancy may decrease.

FITNESS, ENERGY, AND LONGEVITY

One thing is certain. Fitness, energy, and longevity all go hand in hand. In fact, very rarely, if ever, will you see a centenarian who is overweight. The fitter you are the more energy you will have and the more active and energetic you will be next year and the next decade. Your energy is not a function of your age. I'll never forget the time that one of my patients came up to me after his thirtieth birthday and said, "Dr. Plasker, I have been exhausted ever since I turned thirty." A few hours later I had another patient come in who was in his early eighties and he was bouncing around the office like a fireplug. I asked him where he got all his energy and he said to me, "I just had a great workout, a great adjustment, and I am ready to go." He was not limited by his age and you shouldn't be either.

QUALITY YEARS VS. QUANTITY OF YEARS

The number of quality years you live will be determined in large part by your fitness level. If you want to be able to move when you are eighty, ninety, or 100 and beyond, then exercise your mobility now. And make it a priority. Keep your heart healthy now and you will enjoy a healthier heart as you age. Keep your spine healthy and well-adjusted now and you will enjoy flexibility and healthy nerve supply in your later years. Keep your muscles strong now and you will have the freedom to be more active as you age. Living quality years doesn't necessarily ensure a greater quantity of years, but it will ensure greater health and vitality every day along the way.

So many times in my travels I have heard people say, "I don't want to live to be 100. In fact, I don't know if I want to make it to eighty or ninety." Well, you may not have a choice. Remember, today's centenarians didn't want to and didn't plan for it. They never asked for it. You have their genes. Are you willing to adjust your lifestyle so that you make the most of every day along the way? And think about this: If not 100, what's your number? When do you want to pass on? Is it age seventy-three? How about eighty-one, eighty-seven, or ninety-two? If you were active, healthy, and enjoying your life, why would you want your life to come to an end? Unfortunately, we have a skewed view of what our later years could be like because the current ailing nursing home generation was blindsided by their longevity. Their fate is not a result of their age; it's because they didn't prepare for their longevity with a healthy lifestyle. Few people prepared their bodies for the marathon that would take them past age 100.

MAXIMIZE YOUR GENETIC POTENTIAL

I wonder what our true genetic potential really is. Today's centenarians, one of the fastest-growing segments of our population, are outliving their life expectancy by a mind-boggling fifty years. This means that 100 years ago, when this generation was born, their scientific life expectancy was only fifty years. This is a staggering five-decade increase in life span for a generation who grew up in an era of unhealthy foods, smoking (or breathing in secondhand smoke), processed foods, lack of fitness, industrial pollutants, and intense manual labor. In the so-called Blue Zones, which have been written about in other books related to longevity, we see populations that have lived a lifestyle that is more physically active, more connected to nature, eating healthier foods, and who value a close-knit social circle. These are all the qualities that we discuss in The 100 Year Lifestyle.

Will we ever really know the possibilities for human life expectancy? One thing is for sure: If you keep yourself fit and healthy, you will maximize your own innate potential and enjoy quality years along the way. I recently read some articles about the potential life expectancy being 150 years. Is this really that far-fetched? This is only fifty years more than how long people are living today, the same difference between today's life span and the life expectancy 100 years ago. Some scientists are even making claims that we might be able to live one thousand years! The purpose of this book and fitness plan is to help you maximize the expression of your innate potential today so that you can make the most of your personal journey in life, however long that journey may be, living quality years every day while avoiding a decaying and deteriorating future.

JUST LIKE THE PROS

Whether you're just getting started on your ESS program or you're deep into it already, you might be surprised to hear you have something in common with some of the world's most elite athletes. Well, you do. Just like those riding the grueling Tour de France or those squaring off against a ninety-five-mile-an-hour fastball in a major league ball game, it is important to focus on your Endurance, Strength, and Structure.

In the early 1990s when I was practicing on Peachtree Road in Atlanta, my chiropractic office was located one mile up the road from the Ritz Carlton Hotel. Many of the employees became lifetime patients of my practice when they learned about the importance of keeping their spine healthy through the educational programs that we provided. It just made sense to them and they loved the results. They were so excited about how much better, younger, and healthier they felt that, before I knew it, they started to refer many of their hotel guests to my practice for care. This was a lot of fun because their guests included people who were rock stars, royalty, and professional athletes. I will never forget the time when I got called to adjust Isiah Thomas prior to an NBA playoff game. When I got to the hotel with my portable adjusting table, I was excited to see all the television cameras there interviewing Isiah by the pool. I set up my adjusting table and took care of him while they proceeded to film his adjustment for my first-ever national television appearance. It was exciting to get the calls from my colleagues and friends around the country expressing their enthusiasm at seeing this famous athlete receive his chiropractic adjustment. It was even more exciting to see these athletes and entertainers respond to the care and enjoy the experience.

Today, many professional sports teams and top-level athletes include the three elements of the ESS model as an important part of their overall health and wellness plan. I recently spoke to my good friend and colleague, Dr. Jeff Spencer, an attending doctor of chiropractic to some of the top athletes in the world, including PGA winners and a World Series MVP. Dr. Spencer is also the author of the book *Turn It Up*. He has devoted his Web site www.jeffspencer .com to ideas that mirror many of the principles of The 100 Year Lifestyle. His results are well documented and reflected in the success of the athletes he has cared for who have competed in a collective thirty-four world sporting events, including the Tour de France and national and Olympic championships in a variety of different sports. Dr. Spencer knows that *your* body, like those of dominant professionals in their sports, has an amazing ability to heal itself and express its full potential if there is no interference and you keep your ESS in shape. If you stay balanced and keep your structure intact, your spine and body aligned, and your lifestyle balanced, it will make a huge difference in your health and performance. He continues to be sought after for his workout recovery tips and specific techniques for helping the top athletes in the world reach peak performance levels.

Dr. Spencer stresses having a well-balanced, fully integrated personal and professional health management program that covers all the elements of the ESS rather than just one or two. His experience tells him that when a person has devoted too much time in preparation to one area and has not devoted time to the others, there is no way that person can consistently be a top performer—professional and recreational athletes alike. When their spine and nervous system, key body systems, life, and athletic training are out of balance, there are consequences that compromise the level of performance that they can achieve. All of the facets of The 100 Year Lifestyle Workout are equally critical to reaching and maintaining maximum performance and optimal health.

Dr. Spencer was, and is, an athlete himself. He was a Team USA cyclist in the 1972 Munich Olympics. After graduate school, he went on to consult professional athletes in an effort to help them achieve a top level of performance. He eventually went back to chiropractic college for his Doctor of Chiropractic degree because he wanted to work on the athletes' performance and conditioning, as well as placing a major focus on rapid recovery, injury prevention, and management.

One of his greatest successes is his contribution to helping the United States teams achieve eight consecutive Tour de France victories. Dr. Spencer is clear that The 100 Year Lifestyle principles of Endurance, Strength, and Structure are an important part of these athletes' success. In fact, many of the practices that he utilizes to help athletes recover quickly from injuries and perform at their highest level address these elements. He makes every effort to remove all of the interferences in the body that get in the way of peak performance, and he remains one of the top innovators in the chiropractic world.

You too can apply many of the ESS principles that the top athletes use through The 100 Year Lifestyle Workout.

Professional football and basketball teams know how important the three components of the ESS are when it comes to their athletes performing at their highest level. Many of these top athletes get their endurance and strength training on the practice field and in the weight room while their adjustments keep their structure, spine and nervous system healthy. Dr. Greg Kempf from Cleveland, Ohio has been providing chiropractic care for the Cleveland Browns since 1999 and the Cleveland Cavaliers for the past five seasons. He regularly travels with the Browns and occasionally with the Cavs. On game day it is not uncommon for Dr. Kempf to adjust 35 of the 55 members of the team prior to the game. This ritual is commonplace in locker rooms for quite a few teams, and many of their highest profile players receive regular chiropractic care as a part of their training and their lifestyle.

OLYMPIAN COMES BY IT HONESTLY

It's fair to say Dr. Terry Schroeder comes by his profession as a doctor of chiropractic honestly. If you count the fourth generation nephews, there are sixty-six chiropractors in this Olympian and Olympic coach's family. In fact, he doesn't know life without a healthy structure. He has photos of himself being examined and gently adjusted by his chiropractor father at the

ripe old age of two days (the birth process can be very traumatic to a baby's spine).

Over the years, Dr. Schroeder tried many different sports. He excelled at most and he attributes that to the fact that he grew up with his body in perfect balance. By age eight, he was ranked second in the country in a competitive backstroke event. At ages ten through fourteen he hit the fields, trying both baseball and football. By high school though, he found his way into the water again for his dream sport—water polo.

The sport requires tremendous endurance and strength, but most important, a solid and healthy structure. He knew while he was competing how lucky he'd been to have received early chiropractic care and weekly adjustments, encouraged by his father—a habit that to this day continues.

One of the areas in which Dr. Schroeder far outpaced his teammates was his resistance level. It was higher than the rest of the crowd. Many of them had to stay out of the water because they fell ill, but he rarely got sick. And he was able to train at a much higher level as a result. In fact, Dr. Schroeder went his entire career without a major injury.

And that was some career. To this day he is the only five-time Olympian in United States Water Polo—four times making the team as an athlete and once as a coach, though he only competed in the water three times. He made the team in 1980 and was devastated when the Americans boycotted the games, robbing him of a fourth competition. He returned with a vengeance in 1984.

ESS Story: Ray Lankford

Ray is a professional baseball success story. After junior college in Modesto, California, in 1987, he was drafted by the St. Louis Cardinals in the third round, hitting the minors in Springfield, Illinois. He hopped around to a few different cities and spent a season playing winter ball in Puerto Rico, rising through the ranks to Triple A. He was finally called up to the majors in August of 1990, where he spent more than ten years playing for the St. Louis Cardinals and almost four more years playing for the San Diego Padres. He watched many other players with talent not achieve the success he was able to enjoy. Week after week, season after season, the number of players with longevity, durability, and staying power dwindled.

With fourteen seasons and one All-Star Game, Ray was a standout in his sport. He was one of the guys who made it, and his career had longevity. Just getting to the majors alone was an accomplishment. He had talent, but he had something else. He had the skill and understanding that he needed to take care of his body if he wanted to play for the long haul. Talent alone didn't carry him—he had the work ethic, or should I say, the workout ethic, as well.

I recently had an opportunity to interview Ray at the International Chiropractors Association Symposium on Physical Fitness and Sports. Ray was there with his chiropractor Dr. Gerald Mattia, who attracts some of the top athletes in the world to his Orlando, Florida, practice. Ray applied many of The 100 Year Lifestyle's ESS principles to his success as an athlete. His endurance came from his challenging cardio workouts. He and a buddy would crank the treadmill up as fast as it would go and alternate doing thirty-second sprints for ten sets, with thirty-second breaks. He believes the endurance he built up gave him the stamina to endure the long baseball seasons and his marathon career.

Professional baseball players work their

Just like how they could not get enough of the Olympics and the Olympic spirit, many of the athletes could not get enough of the chiropractic care that was being provided for them. They used the care to balance their structure, eliminate nerve pressure, reduce their recovery time and maximize their energy, and it became a key element in their success. Athletes who had chiropractic care were finding a natural edge that some others received from performance-

strength as well. Ray's strength came from working out with light weights, but with lots of reps and explosive movement. He chose lighter weights so that he didn't bulk up, and therefore he was able to maintain his flexibility.

Ray also attributes much of the skill and durability of his game to the care he gave his structure, spine, and nervous system. When he was young, he didn't understand why people had lower back pain or why they went to see a chiropractor, but as he aged, and began feeling the impact of his age, he started to pay attention to his alignment. He started getting spinal adjustments regularly and found it sharpened all aspects of his game. He thought often about how much strain swinging a bat put on his back because of all the twisting. The adjustments kept his spine balanced, sharpened his swing, and even helped his vision so he could line up the bat with the ball. He noticed a difference in everything he did when his body was aligned and balanced. He tracked the ball faster in the field and his recovery time in general was quicker. Whenever he incorporated structure into his training to complete the ESS, he felt better about his game because he knew that everything in his body was aligned, balanced, and firing on all cylinders.

It was the combination of all three—Endurance, Strength, and Structure—that kept him going as he aged and took his performance to a new level. He witnessed his body's response to the ESS concept in a way he didn't understand when he was first starting out in the sport. With his experience and knowledge growing, he continues to keep his ESS in shape even after his baseball career has ended so that he can continue to enjoy the healthy, active quality of life he wants. Unfortunately, many athletes suffer after their retirement due to chronic injuries as well as, for many, an imbalance of their ESS.

enhancing drugs. That's why athletes from many sports and many nations lined up for their adjustments in the Olympic Village.

It wasn't just structure that fueled Dr. Schroeder's edge. While he was training, Dr.

Schroeder made the full ESS a critical part of his athletic career, connecting with the endurance and strength aspects of ESS as well. He did, however, struggle with it after the competition ended. Like many athletes post-career, he had no motivation to go out and exercise. As a result, his system grew out of balance. Many athletes struggle when their careers come to an end, losing their identity after spending so many years training. It becomes a mental and physical challenge at times. This was true for Dr. Schroeder—it was the most difficult time of his life. He kept up with his adjustments, but he let the rest slip. He spent two or three years with those out of balance feelings until he got himself back into the endurance and strength training that got him back on track and balanced.

Structure and the Olympics

Dr. Schroeder started somewhat of a trend as an athlete back in the late seventies. His father would travel with him and do his adjustments and other team members would watch. They were impressed because they knew Dr. Schroeder had an advantage during the games, and they were beginning to understand why. One by one, they started asking for help, mostly after injuries. Eventually adjustments became a regular part of their training routine.

The trend toward chiropractic care caught on widely at the Olympics. The amateur athletic world seemed to embrace the need for this type of care because of the demanding nature of their training, as well as their understanding of the mind-body connection, and its relationship to their structural alignment. It was in 1984 that for the first time a chiropractor was officially credentialed by the U.S. Olympic Committee with access to the athletes like any other part of the medical community. In fact, there were

lines to have the adjustments with chiropractors. Athletes became more and more aware of the edge others were receiving and they flocked to structural care so as not to lose out on any natural advantage. Dr. Jan Corwin treated the athletes; he was the only chiropractor credentialed at the time and he worked long hours.

By the time Dr. Schroeder was coaching in 2008, the movement had exploded. There were four additional official chiropractors as part of the U.S. Olympic staff. Today a chiropractor is in charge of the medical unit.

As a coach, Dr. Schroeder believes care for structure is one of the main reasons his water polo team performed so well—making the shift from number nine in the world to number two. Dr. Schroeder fully embraces the ESS principles of The 100 Year Lifestyle. He teaches the ESS elements to younger and older athletes alike, and encourages them to live The 100 Year Lifestyle to remain healthy and improve their athletic performance.

Many high-level female athletes are also embracing the ESS principles of The 100 Year Lifestyle Workout. Kerri Walsh, the two-time Olympic gold medalist in beach volleyball, told me in a recent interview that she believes that the balance of these three elements are an important factor in her training and her success. Her workouts on the court are cardiovascular in nature and build her endurance. Off the court she does Pilates, plyometrics, and strength-training techniques that give her the added punch she needs for an overhead spike. She also takes care of her structure through chiropractic care and other holistic techniques to balance her spine and keep her muscles strong and flexible. Kerri considers the structural element of her fitness routine to be an important factor that separates her from the pack.

At the age of thirty, Kerri feels like her best performances are ahead of her, and not behind her. Through her commitment to mastering her body and mind, she feels like she can continue to get better at her fitness and her sport. As a big fan of hers, I am looking forward to watching her skills and her legacy grow.

Lauren Wenger, a silver medalist with the women's Olympic water polo team in 2008, and member of USC's national championship team in 2003, also incorporates all three elements of the ESS model into her training and has done so for years. For endurance training she swims four times a week for thirty to forty-five minutes, maintaining her heart rate at Olympic level. After her swimming sessions, she goes into the weight room with her team for strength training, and for her structure, she sees her chiropractor regularly to keep her spine and nervous system aligned and balanced. There have been times when she was injured that she would require three or four adjustments per week, while going less frequently when she was not injured or when her training was less intense. According to Lauren, "You've got to take care of your body and make sure it is aligned and healthy. When you feel something is out of balance, you should take the steps to correct it before it gets worse." This is great advice from some of the top athletes in the world.

Finding a highly qualified professional that understands your goals, and building a team that you trust, can make all the difference in getting the results you want. You can find a 100 Year Lifestyle Provider by going to www.100yearlifestyle.com.

REVERSING YOUR FAMILY HISTORY

People ask me all the time, "What do I do if heart disease runs in my family, or cancer runs in my family?" When I reviewed the top ten leading causes of death in men and women for *The 100 Year Lifestyle* it was very clear that these diseases, while having a genetic component to them, can be prevented through lifestyle. We have become very quick to blame our destiny on our genes. This is an irresponsible choice for us to make. What is responsible is to maximize the health and vitality of your genetics through healthy lifestyle choices. In my corporate and public speeches worldwide, I will always tell the audience, "Raise your hand if your parents or grandparents lived longer than their parents or grandparents." Inevitably 90 percent of the room raises their hands. Living a healthy lifestyle will help you push off those diseases in your history far into the future and maybe even prevent them from happening at all. Living the lifestyle is your responsibility. Learn the Health Care Hierarchy: self-care first, health care second, and crisis care last. When it comes to fitness, self-care and health care will keep you in excellent condition by maintaining your weight, maintaining a healthy metabolism, keeping your heart and circulatory system healthy, your elimination system healthy, and your nervous system firing on all cylinders to optimize the expression of your genes. If you are already in crisis, you can improve your health by making your self-care and health care a priority again while you also focus on healing.

QUALITY OF LIFE VS. CRISIS MOTIVATION

Which one will you choose? Don't wait for a crisis to get your ESS in shape! It's either going to be personal training and a lifestyle of fitness or it's going to be cardiac rehab. You make the choice. They are almost exactly the same except one happens before a heart attack and one happens after a heart attack.

Feeling Older Than Your Age

Here are two significant questions. Write down your answers and then revisit these questions in thirty days.

Question 1: How old are you?
Question 2: How old do you feel?

If you feel older than your age, then you are depriving yourself of a level of quality that you should be enjoying in your life. If you feel your age, you are also depriving yourself of a level of quality that you should be enjoying in your life. You can and should feel younger than your chronological age. How you feel is in great part determined by your energy. If you are overweight and out of shape, then your body is using excess energy just to maintain your current level of survival. If you are sick or suffering from chronic injuries that have not been cared for properly, these require energy just for survival.

Your newfound energy and youthful feeling has to come from somewhere. The Law of Conservation of Energy states that energy can neither be created nor destroyed, but it can be redistributed. Fatty foods require more energy to digest. Why do we get tired when we get the flu or the common cold? Because our body's natural energy gets redirected toward having to heal. When you adjust your lifestyle, your everyday survival requires minimal energy so that all of your excess energy now becomes freed up and can be applied to creative expression, meaningful work, volunteerism, your relationships, hobbies, and involvement in things that matter to you. This is why this high-energy fitness plan is so meaningful. It is so much more than fitness. You will be amazed at how much younger you feel when you free up your energy to engage in the things that you love.

THE POWER OF CHOICE

Life is full of choice, so much so that it can sometimes be overwhelming. There are so many fitness options out there to choose from. Drive down the road in most towns in the country, and you'll see a barrage of food choices, ranging from fast food to slow food, to poor-quality food, to food in a fun environment and food in a dirty environment. The options are almost unlimited. When you go to the grocery store to buy food for your home, you'll also notice the abundance of options. There are grocery stores that specialize in unhealthy processed food and there are grocery stores that specialize in nutritious healthy food. Even in the same grocery store you have many of these options combined. From this point forward I am going to invite you to wake up to choice and become conscious of everything that you think, eat, and do. You'll make The 100 Year Lifestyle your own, which will give you the power of choice on your side.

Food and fitness go hand in hand when it comes to choice. The fitness options that are available to you today are so plentiful that they might even be overwhelming. Choose not to be overwhelmed and get on the path.

There are fitness centers that you can go to that have everything under one roof, from first-class strength-training machines and endurance-training equipment to group fitness classes, basketball courts, racquetball courts, and swimming pools. These fitness meccas serve a purpose by providing numerous options, highly trained staff, and a fitness environment where you could never get bored. There are also boutique fitness centers that usually have higher fees and focus on individual attention for people who desire serious support.

Home fitness options range from exercise DVDs and dumbbells to complete home gym systems for rooms of any size and shape.

The WORST choice you can make: choosing nothing. With so many options out there today it can be easy to simply not choose anything because you don't know where to start. It could also be easy to get in a rut of doing the same old things you have always done. It's time to become conscious and wake up to the power of choice and begin living your ideal 100 Year Lifestyle. Because we have so many options available to us, I believe we take the power of choice for granted and this keeps us from getting over the hump or truly living to our full potential.

CHOOSE TO LIKE THE THINGS THAT ARE GOOD FOR YOU

I was talking to a client recently who was having challenges with her health, and she was looking to make some changes. She described all the things that she liked to eat and all the foods that she enjoyed, saying that everything she liked was bad for you. I said to her the same thing I will say to you: Choose to like the things that are good for you.

Whether it is healthy food, or fitness as a way of life, it is important for you to choose to like the things that are good for you. Eating things that are good for you makes you feel good. Healthy foods keep you regularly going to the bathroom so that you do not feel bloated. They provide you with the fuel through good nutrition to give you more energy and mental focus, and they keep you slender so that you like what you see when you look in the mirror. When you choose to eat the things that you do, understanding the power of choice, don't just choose for taste. Taste is just one element. The other benefits of the food you put in your mouth should be equally important. The good news is that there are so many options out there that also taste good, once you get used to the slightly different way the food tastes you will begin to enjoy it.

The same is true for movement. Wake up to the power of choice and choose to move rather than be sedentary or a couch potato. Choose to go to the gym or to go for a workout rather than the immobile alternatives. In *The 100 Year Lifestyle* we talked about the Dominant Energy Patterns that people get into, which include destructive patterns, survival patterns, complacency patterns, comfort patterns, and human potential patterns. Through the power of choice, you can decide to change your overall energy pattern from survival to human potential and from complacency and comfort to your own human potential pattern. Begin by having a 100 percent conscious day and become aware of everything that you think, eat, and do. When you catch

yourself reaching for unhealthy foods or using unhealthy movement patterns or not moving much at all, do what we call "The Midstream Catch"; stop yourself right in the middle of your destructive and unhealthy act and exercise the power of choice. Decide in that moment that you will choose your own human potential pattern. In the beginning you may find that you do 100 midstream catches a day, and as you make these choices in your new lifestyle you may only need to do this once a week or once a month. There is no shortcut to this process.

THE THREE LIFE-CHANGING PRINCIPLES AND YOUR 100 YEAR LIFESTYLE WORKOUT

As you implement this fitness plan, keep in mind the three life-changing principles of The 100 Year Lifestyle. Life-changing principle #1: Change is easy; thinking about change is hard. It's easier to be fit than it is to be fat. It's easier to be healthy than it is to be sick. It's easier to be forty pounds lighter than to be forty pounds heavier. It's easier to eat healthy than it is to go through life living from crisis to crisis because you are overweight. It's easier to say no to sugar than it is to hate yourself for being out of control. Draw a line in the sand.

I remember, when I was forty pounds heavier than I am now, I needed to draw a line in the sand with chocolate. Chocolate would talk to me from 100 miles away. In fact it would scream at me from 100 miles away. When I was undecided and uncommitted to my new lifestyle, I would listen to the chocolate and it would get the best of me when it would say "eat me." However, when I committed to the change, the chocolate stopped talking to me, and when it did talk to me, I won. I remember one time when I was on a ski trip with my brothers, Jordan and Noel, to celebrate my brother Noel's fortieth birthday. We were at a beautiful resort in Snow Bird, Utah. I remember walking into the hotel room and immediately noticing a fifteen-foot hallway leading into the bedroom. Even though I could not see the bed, I knew there was something waiting for me there. Can you guess what it was? You're right. It was chocolate, fine chocolate. I couldn't even see the chocolate on the bed but I knew it was there and I immediately went right up to it, told it to shut up, crumbled it up, and threw it in the garbage.

Having the edge and drawing the line in the sand is going to make the changes you are about to commit to much easier to follow through on. Remember, life-changing principle #1: Change is easy; thinking about change is hard.

Life-changing principle #2: Change comes one choice at a time. Think progress, not perfection. Just like it wasn't the first cookie, the first beer, or the first cigarette that may have started your health decline, it won't be the first workout, the first healthy meal, the first personal training session, or the first spinal adjustment that makes you healthy again. It will be the lifestyle that makes you healthy. In spite of all the media hype about our nation's obesity and the reality shows dedicated to weight loss, I believe that our focus on weight loss is responsible for our individual roller coaster ride and our nation's health decline.

In a society so committed to winning on every level from youth and professional sports to relationships and business, it is no wonder we struggle so much with our weight when the entire focus is on loss. I believe this creates a personal state of deprivation that keeps people from staying committed to a healthy lifestyle. Constantly thinking about what you can't have, then resenting the fact that you can't have it, will eventually only make you want it more, and for many people this leads to periods of uncontrollable consumption. Living the Lifestyle and becoming healthy is about so much more than weight loss.

We gain so much from living a healthy lifestyle. We gain more energy, a greater sense of vitality, increased personal confidence, and a feeling of being sexy, which is another one of those things that we all crave. We also gain a better quality of life and an opportunity for greater quality of life as we age. When you commit to this lifestyle, you make choices every day regarding the food that you eat, the places

Draw a line in the sand with the three life-changing principles of The 100 Year Lifestyle:

Change Principle #1: Change is easy. Thinking about change is hard.

Change Principle #2: Change happens one choice at a time. Think progress, not perfection.

Change Principle #3: Approach change with your ideal 100 Year Lifestyle in mind.

you shop, and the way that you move, exercise, and take care of your body, mind, and spirit to ensure that you fill your marathon life with quality years. With every 100 Year Lifestyle choice you make, you will gain confidence and build momentum. Remember, nobody is perfect, so if you get off track with a bad meal or a missed workout, this life-changing principle will get you back on track with your choices.

Life-changing principle #3: If you are going to make a change, make it with your ideal 100 Year Lifestyle in mind. Another reason why people struggle when they try to begin a fitness plan is because they lack an exciting motivation. Make the reasons for your lifestyle changes compelling. You are not going to lose weight for the rest of your life unless you gain it back over and over again, which means you're always losing weight. This isn't compelling. It's exhausting.

What are some compelling reasons for you to change your lifestyle? Do you want to live a healthy, drug-free life? Do you want to wake up energized every day? Do you want to feel more confident during job interviews, sales calls, or meeting your new life partner?

I've learned some interesting things about what causes people to begin a fitness program. I was recently invited to be the keynote speaker at the Gold's Gym Body Transformation Challenge in Newburgh, New York. I asked the head trainer, Dave Kenyon, what are some of the most common reasons people come in and what causes them to commit to a gym membership and personal training? I was surprised to learn that people who are going through a divorce or just got divorced make up a large percentage of new exercisers. Why? Many people, when they get in a committed relationship, let themselves go from a health standpoint and through their relationship crisis they realize that if they want to get in a new relationship they are more likely to find one if they are healthier. This causes them to commit to changing their lifestyle and working out.

One of the exercises in *The 100 Year Lifestyle* is to set 100 year goals. Make your own personal bucket list of things that you want to do before you die. Keep in mind, you're going to have to be fit to complete this checklist and enjoy yourself while you do them. But living the 100 Year Lifestyle is so much more than

Compelling Questions to Create Compelling Reasons to Change

Would that be a compelling reason to stop procrastinating and get you to change your lifestyle?

Are you ready to look and feel younger and healthier?

Do you want to regain youthful energy?

Do you want to travel the world no matter what your age?

Are you sick of being in pain?

Do you want to be able to enjoy being outside, hiking, or walking, not just today but throughout your lifetime?

What would you like to become an expert in over the next decade?

Will you enjoy it more if you are fit?

How would your relationship improve right now if you committed to changing your lifestyle before you get in a relationship crisis?

checking things off a list. It's about being able to enjoy the things that you love for a lifetime. How important is being fit and healthy to help you accomplish and enjoy your eighty, ninety, or 100 years and beyond? The 100 Year Lifestyle is actually a massive paradigm shift in consciousness while also being a strategic way to live your lifestyle.

Make a list of the compelling reasons to stay on track with your lifestyle. Think of things that will motivate you to make changes because they have your ideal 100 Year Lifestyle in mind.

EXHAUSTING VS. HIGH-ENERGY TRAINING

Remember, exercise and fitness should give you energy. It should not be exhausting. If you are one of those people who gets exhausted by exercise, then you are doing something wrong. Maybe you're not taking in enough calories and this makes you tired. Maybe you're not eating frequently enough and your blood sugar is on a roller coaster. It could be that you're eating the wrong kinds of foods or it may be that the type of exercise that you are doing is not the right type of exercise for you given your age, your current health condition, or previous injuries that you have had. Either way, if you are already exercising but you are tired all the time, stop blaming exercise for your lack of energy. We will discuss healthy eating patterns and different styles of high-energy training throughout this book. For now, it's important that you look to other areas for the source of your exhaustion and begin making some changes to keep your energy state naturally high.

Live Long and Strong—Personal Energy Inventory

When you get your ESS in shape, you will feel energized. You can begin to increase your energy now by having a 100 percent conscious day, taking note of all the things that zap your energy in a negative way. On the other hand also take notice of the things that give you energy. From a fitness perspective, maybe you are doing too much endurance or cardio training and not enough strength training. Strength training can increase metabolism and give you more energy. If you are one of those people who don't eat breakfast, change your pattern and start your day with a healthy breakfast from one of the breakfast recipes in this book. Or, if you go more than three or four hours without eating every day, it could drain your energy, so start incorporating healthy snacks periodically throughout the day and choose from the healthy snacks list. This will stabilize your blood sugar. If you normally don't eat before you exercise, have a protein shake or bar thirty minutes prior to your workout and eat a healthy meal within two hours after your workout. Begin to experiment with different foods and the timing of your meals to find the high energy human potential pattern that is uniquely yours. The 100 Year Lifestyle Workout is about living the highest quality life every day of your life for 100 years and beyond. There is nothing depriving about it.

Throughout this book you will learn a lot of the things that you should be doing to get the most out of your workouts and get in the best shape of your life. It is also important to know what not to do. In the next chapter, you will learn how to avoid the top sixteen fitness mistakes that people make as they age. Avoiding these pitfalls will keep you on a steady and consistent course while preventing unnecessary pain and injury along the way. It's time for you to embrace your longevity and the healthy lifestyle that will help you enjoy it.

CHAPTER TWO:

Avoid the Top Sixteen Fitness Mistakes People Make as They Age

Since you have made it this far, let's start you out on the right path and avoid the setbacks that plague so many people who want to get fit and healthy but get derailed unnecessarily because they made beginner mistakes. One of the keys to your success in this program will be gaining momentum along the way, and if you follow this plan and avoid the hiccups that can occur, your consistency will keep you inspired and motivated naturally.

We are about to review the top sixteen avoidable mistakes people make when they begin a fitness plan. If you are a new exerciser, or if you are just getting back into fitness after a decade or two layoff, please review all of these carefully because any one can set you back with injuries or the frustration that comes with a lack of results.

If you are an experienced exerciser review them anyway, because avoiding these mistakes can help you break through a plateau that may be discouraging you and keeping you from taking your health and fitness up a notch. Take note of the specific mistakes that you feel are more directly related to you, and take action to ensure that you do what is necessary to avoid them.

1. DOING IT FOR SOMEONE ELSE

Congratulations on making it this far through *The 100 Year Lifestyle Workout*—you're obviously motivated. To guarantee that you stay on your path, you must do this for the right reason. You have to do it for you. What's often unique about people who are forty, fifty, or sixty years old who begin a fitness plan is that it's the first time in decades they're putting themselves first. Many of us have spent years taking care of our spouse first, our children first, our parents first, and we have let ourselves go in the process. It's time to put yourself at the top of your list. Put your fitness first. And do it for you.

I was recently flying to California to deliver a 100 Year Lifestyle seminar to a group of doctors. As I watched the safety video that I had seen many times before, I noticed something important. The video mentioned that if a sudden change in cabin pressure occurred, oxygen masks would appear. We were instructed to place our own mask on first, before assisting our children. This would ensure that we received the oxygen we needed to be better able to assist the people we love. Your fitness will be like your oxygen. If you are fit, healthy, and happy, you will have more energy to be a better spouse, partner, parent, or child. You are worth it.

I was talking to one of our clients recently who happens to be a doctor, and he was telling me that he woke up one day and realized that he was nearly 100 pounds overweight. It took the scale for him to realize how badly he'd taken care of himself. Everyone around him was telling him to lose weight and take better care of himself and, in fact, that he should practice what he'd been preaching to his patients. He had tried many times to practice what he preached, but because he hadn't committed to doing it for himself, he never followed through. It's a good lesson for everyone—to make sure you understand why you're changing your life. Whether you're in crisis or simply want to improve your quality of life, make a self-motivated choice to do it for you. You'll be the one to benefit from your workouts. You will be the one who sleeps in your bed, looks in the mirror, walks up the stairs, or lays in a hospital bed or nursing facility. The self-care component of the Health Care Hierarchy was written for you especially. Remember, nobody can sweat for you. That's just something you are going to have to do for yourself. Do it for you.

2. STARTING TOO FAST

One of the most common mistakes people make when they're forty, fifty, and sixty and they start a fitness program again or try to break through a plateau is that they start out too fast. They remember the days when they used to be able to run for an hour, do a back flip, or sprint the forty-yard dash in less than five seconds. They try to reproduce that level of fitness instantaneously.

Guess what? Attempting to move like you did when you were twenty is a bad idea.

If you've let your body go and you've gotten yourself way out of shape, get back into it slowly. Embrace The 100 Year Lifestyle Workout with the mindset of life-changing principle number two: Change comes one choice at a time. Think progress not perfection. Just like it wasn't the first cookie or piece of cake that got you into your current health predicament and packed on the extra pounds, your first workout is not going to be the one that changes your life. Don't try to lose all your excess weight from one workout. Change will come one choice at a time with progress rather than perfection as you consistently create your own healthy, customized 100 Year Lifestyle plan.

Starting too fast can lead to injuries that slow you down and set you back. If you're out of shape, injuries may require a longer healing time, so do not overdo it. Begin these workouts with a pace that's comfortable for you. Get a week or two under your belt and then begin to increase the three key elements of The 100 Year Lifestyle Workout, which are Frequency, Intensity, and Duration.

Frequency—How Often You Exercise

You should be exercising between four and six days per week. You will vary the intensity, duration, and focus of your workouts on these days, but you will be working out on some level and at some capacity four to six times a week. When you try to reverse a decade of an unhealthy lifestyle in the first week and exercise intensely every day, you are starting too fast. Do a little bit each day and train yourself to get in the habit of exercising and eating healthy. Developing the habit is extremely important to changing your lifestyle, so consistency matters. Give your body recovery time so that you avoid injuries and look forward to your workouts.

Intensity—The Number of Calories You Burn Per Hour of Exercise

As you improve your fitness you'll increase your intensity, which will make your workouts much more efficient. A low-intensity walk may burn 350 calories per hour whereas a high-intensity elliptical session, fitness class, hike, or run might burn up to 750 calories per hour. Starting with high-intensity activities can lead to injuries, such as pulled muscles or an acute spinal injury. This doesn't need to happen to you, and starting too fast can create frustration by slowing you down in the long run. When you are consistent with your frequency, you will build the stamina to increase your intensity. This can occur within your first two weeks. Varying your intensity will be a source of motivation for you and will inspire you as you see your progress.

Duration—The Length of Time You Work Out

The more fit you become the longer the duration of your workouts can be. We have laid out a fitness plan for beginner, intermediate, and advanced exercisers to get your ESS in shape, keep your ESS in shape, and take your ESS to the next level. Varying the Frequency, Intensity, and Duration will ensure a healthy experience and maximize your results.

As your stamina increases and your body requires less rest, you can increase the frequency of your workouts by going to the gym five times a week instead of four times a week. You can go twice a day instead of once a day. You can increase your intensity by raising your heart rate higher and burning more calories during your workouts. It's important to monitor your progress, especially if you have a past history of health problems. You can also increase the length of your workouts as your stamina improves one choice at a time, one workout at a time, with progress not perfection.

As time goes on you will gain confidence in your body and your mind as you enjoy the newfound health that comes with your commitment to making exercise and fitness a part of your lifestyle.

3. BEING CRISIS MOTIVATED

People remain on the roller coaster of weight loss and weight gain primarily because they are motivated by crisis only. Unfortunately, for many people, tight pants or severe physical symptoms are the impetus for trying to lose weight, instead of a decision to commit to a fit and healthy lifestyle.

In *The 100 Year Lifestyle,* we explored the difference between people who are crisis motivated and people who are quality of life motivated. When it comes to fitness, people who are crisis motivated require some type of wake-up call to get them to do the things they know are good for them. Maybe they have a special occasion to go to and they go to their closet, attempt to put on their clothes, and they don't fit. Maybe it's the fact that they wake up one day with excruciating back pain because they have been carrying around an extra load for a long time, which is putting unnecessary strain on their spine and nerve system. Maybe they choose to work out because their blood pressure or their blood sugar skyrockets to the top of the charts.

Remember, this crisis motivated mentality of "if it ain't broke don't fix it" was the philosophy of the nursing home generation. Today's centenarians were blindsided by their extended life spans and adopted this attitude as a lifestyle. Unfortunately, they defined "broke" as serious, life-threatening disease or excruciating pain and did not make healthy choices and healthy living their way of life. We're getting the advance notice that our parents and grandparents never received: Life is a marathon and not a sprint, and we should adopt a lifestyle that is quality of life motivated rather than crisis motivated to ensure that we live our best lives every day. In *The 100 Year Lifestyle* we define "broke" as being out of balance.

The problem with crisis motivation as your driving force for healthy decisions and choices is that your lifestyle will get out of balance constantly. Living from crisis to crisis can become a way of life, a habit.

Healthy people rarely get sick. Overweight, unhealthy people with unhealthy lifestyles are more susceptible to life-threatening illnesses as they age, such as heart disease, stroke, cancer, and diabetes. They also compromise their quality of life every day along the way.

Crisis motivation may be enough to get you started in a lifestyle of health and wellness, but it will not be enough to keep you there. At some point your motivation must become quality of life driven. If your goal is to lose weight, what are you going to do when the weight is gone? You're going to need a different motivation. For long-term health, choose quality of life motivation that keeps you healthy, inspires you to get more out of your body, and keeps you on top of your game. You will love the results that come with your new lifestyle.

4. STARVATION DIETS

Hearing my patients and seminar attendees talk about their eating habits always interests me. One of the most common mistakes people make when it comes to food and eating habits is that they starve themselves and deprive their bodies of the calories they need to live an active, healthy, energetic life. The upcoming section on measuring calories will be a huge eye opener for you, and you can get started on this now by going to www.100yearlifestyle.com.

I've always been amazed in my chiropractic practice by the adaptive capabilities of the human body. Every person has within them an innate intelligence, a guiding life-force, that will always do all it can to keep its host alive and in the best shape it can even in the worst circumstances. The negative side of this is that the body will adapt to starvation by slowing down its metabolism. If you binge eat after starving yourself, because your metabolism is slower, your body will store the extra calories as fat to protect you from future episodes of starvation.

It's incredible how the body can adapt. I had a patient in her mid-eighties who was suffering from a thyroid goiter the size of an orange that was bulging out of her neck. She had chosen not to have it removed, and amazingly her body was able to adapt. I have seen numerous pregnant women with their weight gains and weight losses over a nine-month period of time and I'm always fascinated to see how their bodies adapted. Kyle Maynard is a friend and patient of mine who was born with no arms or legs, and yet he was able to adapt and become an incredible high school wrestler and power lifting record holder. Now he runs his own gym, has a bestselling book *No Excuses,* and speaks around the country. I am amazed at how he is able to adapt his lifting style to maximize his strength.

Another patient of mine was, at the time, the world light heavyweight kickboxing champion, and his muscles also adapted to his training. They developed like thick rubber bands, strong, loose, and flexible, which helped him with his martial arts training and world championship run.

Rather than looking at your body and thinking that you are too old, or too fat, or too tired, I propose you take a positive spin on your situation. Marvel at your body's ability to adapt to the way you have taken care of it for the past few years or the past few decades. Your body has adapted to the unhealthy, sedentary, destructive lifestyle habits that you have either consciously or unconsciously chosen. Don't starve yourself because your body will adapt.

Don't just think about losing weight. Don't just think about deprivation. We grow up not wanting to lose at sports, not wanting to lose the debate, and not wanting to lose at anything we try. Nobody wants to lose. Yet when it comes to our health, the first question that we ask someone is, "how much weight have you lost?" This is only half of the equation. If you don't connect to the gains that your new, healthy, ideal 100 Year Lifestyle is bringing to you, you too will find yourself being defeated by the constant deprivation game.

5. WORKING OUT LIKE YOU'RE EIGHTEEN AGAIN

If you are a former athlete, or you used to work out, and have let yourself go, let me remind you that you aren't eighteen anymore despite the fact that you want to be. It's easy to remember how you used to be. Let this be the motivation for your long-term fitness goals, but don't start out like you are eighteen again. When I was in high school, I played football as an offensive guard, and I was into power lifting. At my best I bench pressed 325 pounds and was, as my children would say, "a beast." A few years ago, when I began strength training again, I walked into the gym and there just happened to be 225 pounds on a bench press. I looked at it and thought to myself *what the heck let's give it a shot.* Boy, was I disappointed when I couldn't even lift the bar off of the bench. What a blow to my ego when I remembered being able to do 225 for a dozen reps. Fortunately, I shook it off quickly and found my new starting point with a new Get Your ESS in Shape fitness plan. You'll be able to do the same.

A few years ago I had a patient who was an All-Star high school and college tennis player. Fit and healthy for most of her life, she had quit playing tennis and let herself go by gaining around twenty-five pounds. Working out in a gym or by herself was not really her thing. She loved the competitiveness of tennis and wanted to get back into it. Unfortunately she started too fast and soon learned that diving for a ball in a meaningless match was not a good idea. After a series of adjustments, and then working with

her to keep her structure balanced and her nervous system healthy through a wellness adjustment plan, she got back on the court for the fun of it. Within six months she found her groove and her old-time skills and is enjoying her passion once again. The good news is that her new style of play will enable her to enjoy tennis for the rest of her sensational century.

6. INSUFFICIENT RECOVERY TIME

As you begin your fitness plan, you will get to know your body and learn what your recovery time needs to be. It is not healthy to work out your biceps every day. It is not healthy to run ten miles every day. As you age, cross training becomes more important because you use different muscle groups and keep yourself fit and moving while giving parts of your body time to rest. You will see as we lay out your fitness plan that certain body parts are worked out on specific days while giving alternative days for them to rest. This allows for sufficient recovery time.

7. FAILING TO WARM UP

Stretching and flexibility exercises are one of the most important and underutilized fitness techniques for people of all ages. A proper warm-up and cool-down can help speed recovery time and minimize soreness especially in the beginning. And it's not just middle-age exercisers that neglect to get a stretch in before and after a workout, it's everyone. My son, Cory, plays on a high-level soccer team, Ambush Elite in Alpharetta, Georgia, which at the time of this writing is ranked second in the nation. They are youth partners of West Ham United of the English Premier League which is known for its high-level training as one of the best youth soccer academies in the world.

One of my hobbies is to adjust his team to keep the players' bodies balanced, and their spines and nervous systems healthy. I provide them with complimentary chiropractic care, and I have been doing this for his soccer teams since he was six years old. I love it and so do the kids. It's exciting that his teams have never had a major injury or a player that has missed more than one game due to injury. As most professional athletes will tell you, this is definitely one of the advantages of having a chiropractor as a member of your health care team.

David Eristavi, Cory's current coach and one of the top youth coaches in the nation, insists that his players take ten to fifteen minutes of dynamic warm-ups before practice and ends practice with five to ten minutes of cool-down and stretching. This is important to ensure sufficient recovery time. As a former professional player whose team utilized these techniques along with chiropractic care, he knows the importance of these principles for optimizing the performance and longevity of his players. If you are just starting a fitness program again or you are new to fitness altogether, you will probably get sore in your muscles and in your spine. Soreness is different than being injured. You can speed recovery time with a ten-minute cool-down and stretching routine and keeping your spine well adjusted and balanced.

8. NOT GETTING ENOUGH QUALITY SLEEP

You should be getting between seven and nine hours of quality sleep per night. Your body needs the recovery time that quality sleep brings. Lack of sleep, especially accumulated over time, will lower your energy, make you chronically tired, take away from your ability to concentrate and focus, adversely affect your memory, disconnect you from people and the ability to be present, and over the long haul can make you sick.

Secrets to a Quality Sleep

- A good supportive bed that stabilizes your spine and adjusts to your body as you age

- If your bed does not allow you to vary the firmness of the mattress and/or does not adjust to the contour of your body, don't sleep in it for twenty years.

- Pillows: You must sleep on a pillow that provides triple support and fits the contour of your upper back, neck, and head. As you age, the spinal disks in your neck will deteriorate if they are not aligned properly. Since you probably spend seven to eight hours a night in a bed, having the right kind of support from your pillow can keep your neck aligned and free from nerve pressure. Go to www.100yearlifestyle.com for more information on pillows that provide this kind of support.

ESS Story: David Eristavi

Youth Sports Programs Embrace ESS Principles

David Eristavi is one of the top youth soccer coaches in the country. He was a professional athlete in the Republic of Georgia and the former head coach for the Atlanta Silverbacks. In the Republic of Georgia men at seventy years and older cook for themselves, work in the gardens, and dance. His great grandpa died at 119 years old. At 115 he was riding a horse. David had a left knee meniscus injury when he was younger. His neighbor introduced him to a doctor that adjusted him and in one day he was fixed. That was thirty-six years ago and he's never required surgery.

In my native country of Georgia, people live long lives. As a part of the culture, they follow the principles of Dr. Plasker's 100 Year Lifestyle by doing work that builds their endurance and gives them strength, and they realize the importance of taking care of their structure. I started playing soccer there at a very young age and went on to become a professional soccer player for the Republic of Georgia's national and professional teams.

We were very fortunate that our training took the ESS into account. In Russia fitness is big! We were called the Russian Brazilians we worked so hard. We practiced and performed endurance training that included agility training uniquely focused on developing soccer skills. We performed exercises that helped build our strength in a way that was important for developing our needs on the soccer field, and our coaches knew how important it was to take care of our structure. As professional soccer players we were fortunate to have a team chiropractor to take care of us. The team would fly in our doctor to adjust our spines and balance our bodies so that our nervous systems and muscles were functioning at a very high level. Our players would line up to get their adjustments and truly appreciated that the balance of these three components of the ESS were considered in our care. I believe this balanced fitness plan helped our team stay healthy and contributed greatly to our success. Soccer is a gladiator's game and pain can be relieved quickly with adjustments.

Now as a head soccer coach and program director for some of the most successful youth girls and boys teams in the nation, I have brought many of these principles to my training and coaching techniques. Just as my teammates and I used to line up for our adjustments, our young players also line up

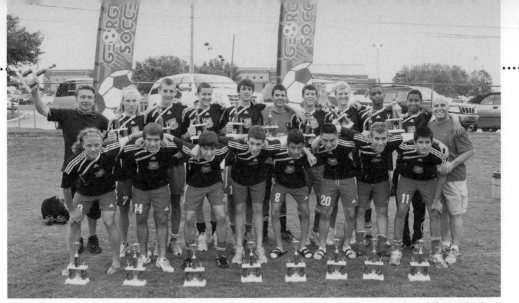

The nationally ranked U-17 Ambush Elite soccer team after winning the 2009 Atlanta Cup. From left to right, back row: Coach David Eristavi, Trevor Greenwald, Stewart Abrahart, Dalton Walsh, Matt Palma, Kevin Quintana, Jeffrey Degen, Chase Reineke, Darion Copeland, Karl Chester, Dr. Eric Plasker. Front row: Josh Boone, Bo Stroup, Ara Amirkhanian, Cory Plasker, Hector Alvarado, Andres Morales, Eric Carrion, Jaime Sanclemente.

for their adjustments, especially prior to the big games. Just last December our under-sixteen boys team, the Ambush Elite, went down to the Disney Showcase Tournament and won our bracket beating several of the top teams in the nation. Our kids got their adjustments prior to every game to ensure that their bodies were in top condition. I believe this made a huge difference for us as it did when we also won the Atlanta Cup and many other games during the season. We finished as one of the top teams in the nation.

Our endurance training during practices gave us the stamina that we needed to compete, while the strength training through specific soccer-style exercises gave us the power that we needed, and the structure kept us aligned and balanced so that the kids could function at their highest level and have the best chance to win. I believe that all youth coaches in all sports should follow the principles of The 100 Year Lifestyle in their training with kids. We have to remember that competitive sports, including soccer in particular, can be brutal on the bodies of these young athletes, and the balance of all three of these elements will not only ensure their success on the field today but also their health and activity for a lifetime. I believe it is very, very important for children to get a good stretch and adjustment to balance their bodies while they are young. As kids get older, they need to stretch their muscles and keep their joints aligned.

Keeping my ESS in balance helped me in my soccer career and still keeps me healthy today, along with good nutrition and a good attitude. It will also help our young athletes heal quickly, prevent injuries, and improve their performance for a lifetime.

Regular exercise through The 100 Year Lifestyle Workout can improve the quality of your sleep dramatically. When you burn energy during your workouts, you will find that your energy throughout your day increases significantly, and you will also find that you begin to sleep like a baby again.

9. IT'S NOT ABOUT THE SIXPACK, UNLESS OF COURSE YOU WANT ONE

For some people, fitness is their life. Their body and the quality of their abs determines the level of their income. This is not true for most of us. For most of us, being fit enables us to enjoy an incredible quality of life. However at the same time you must understand that the abdominal muscles that make up your sixpack are an important part of your core. And for you to be healthy and strong you must have a strong core. There is an entire section in *The 100 Year Lifestyle Workout* called *Going Core Crazy* and, yes, we want you to go core crazy. If you have a strong core, you will be strong everywhere. You will be more durable, you will minimize the possibility of injuries to your spine, and you will look good.

In the United States people spend nearly $100 billion on back-related injuries, many of which could have been prevented with a strong core and a healthy lifestyle. Your core includes your abdominal muscles, your obliques, your hip flexors, your gluteal muscles, and your lower back muscles. When you go core crazy this area of your body, which houses your center of gravity, will be more stable, durable, and stronger. A strong core will improve athletic performance, quickness, and overall strength while also keeping you lean and attractive in a bathing suit. Get excited about the core element of The 100 Year Lifestyle Workout and you may end up with your sixpack anyway.

10. POOR EATING HABITS

If you're trying to get your ESS in shape and you're finding that you take two steps forward and one step backwards, you likely have poor eating habits that are slowing you down. Just like you are changing your fitness habits, it is important to change your eating habits. I was recently talking to a client who was having challenges with her weight and her energy. She knew that her body burned approximately 1,800 calories a day. And she thought that if she starved herself by eating one meal a day she would cut her calories and lose weight. She skipped breakfast every day, had an iceberg lettuce salad for lunch, and then ate whatever she wanted for dinner knowing that she was taking in fewer calories than she was burning. The problem: Throughout the day, her energy was extremely low. She found it difficult to focus and concentrate. Her body went into survival mode because she was starving herself, and she became a slightly smaller version of herself, but she was unhappy with her lifestyle and her weight bounced up and down like a roller coaster. When you eat can be just as important as what you eat. We will provide several options for meal plans later in this book, and you can customize and create your own by going to www.100yearlifestyle.com.

I recently attended a convention where I heard fitness legend, former Mr. Olympia and my colleague, Dr. Franco Colombu, speaking about health and fitness. During the question and answer session, I asked him how he calmed patients' fears about having their muscle turn to fat as they got older. I told him about one of my patients who made a comment to me about how he has seen many big strong athletes lose their muscle and gain lots of fat and he did not want that to happen to him. Dr. Colombu responded by stating that muscle doesn't turn to fat. He explained that these athletes lose their mass because they stop training. Because they stop training, the amount of calories they burn goes down, yet unfortunately many of these athletes continue eating at the same rate as they did when competing. This creates a big calorie surplus, which causes them to gain fat. This may have happened to you if you are a former athlete. It is important to get your eating habits under control and adjust your food intake to your lifestyle.

11. DON'T COMPENSATE PROPERLY FOR PREVIOUS INJURIES

Several years ago I tore my medial collateral ligament and my anterior cruciate ligament, better known as my MCL and ACL. I'll never forget that day. I was skiing with my boys in Lake Louise, Canada, and the last words that my wife, Lisa, said to me before she took off with my daughter Emily were, "be careful; don't hurt yourself." We were careful on the black diamond slopes that we were skiing, but while

we were on a pre-green slope (for you non-skiers this is about the easiest terrain that you can ski or snowboard on), I stopped paying attention for a split second, caught an edge, and felt my knee go pop. I rode down the mountain on a snowmobile, embarrassed for myself and feeling bad that I was going to have to cut my vacation short while everyone else enjoyed the slopes.

I realized through my rehabilitation that I was going to have to change my workouts while I recovered. I rode the stationary bike instead of walking on the treadmill for my endurance training. I used machines for my strength training instead of free weights because I needed the additional support and stability that the machines were able to give me. I got on a corrective adjustment plan with my chiropractor and got adjusted more frequently because all of that limping around was causing my spine to be unbalanced, which in turn affected the pressure on my lower back nerves, which in turn affected my knee. I believe my willingness to adapt my workouts and my self-care and health care was a big part of my speedy recovery. Now I can ski, exercise, hike, and do everything I want to do without any problems.

On the flipside, I have seen countless patients over the years who were unwilling to adapt their fitness plan and their lifestyle as they aged. One in particular was a prominent attorney in town who came to see me after injuring his lower back while he was out for a run. I looked at his x-rays and he had severe deterioration in his lower back and his neck surrounding his bones and his disks. With these chronic vertebral subluxations, spinal injuries with nerve pressure, and osteoarthritis, he was suffering severely at fifty, much too young of an age. Fortunately, he responded extremely well to his chiropractic care and was feeling better and ready to start running again within a few weeks. I told him that based on the condition of his spine, I strongly recommended that he consider a different form of endurance training. I suggested that low-impact training would be a better choice for him given the level of deterioration that he had accumulated in his spine from years of neglect. At first he didn't follow my advice and constantly re-injured his spine. Finally, after re-injuring his back one time too many, he listened, took my advice, and started doing low-impact training. His fitness program began to keep him healthy instead of perpetuating his suffering. The balance of the ESS is

ESS Story: Toby Reece

When Toby Reece was in his mid-twenties, he was in great physical shape and surfed almost every day on some of the largest swells in southern California. He would wait tables at a busy restaurant at night and surf "barrels" in the morning. One weekend while he was helping an elderly neighbor paint his house, he fell off a thirty-foot ladder onto cement. That fall damaged the bottom three vertebrae of his spine and he was lucky to avoid paralysis.

This injury continued to have negative effects on his life just a few years after the trauma. Despite increasing levels of pain, Toby followed a lifelong dream to open a sushi restaurant in Seal Beach, California, not far from his favorite spot for great waves. However, his past began to interrupt his bright future. With three herniated lower back discs, intense sciatica, and decreasing activity levels, he was scheduled to have surgery. The unknown outcome of a risky surgery had the young father considering the sale of his now popular restaurant. The financial impact would be devastating. Between his severe stress and now complete inactivity, he gained over forty pounds while his health quickly declined. The pain was so intense he sought a local chiropractor with the simple expectation of being more comfortable until the surgical date.

What he found in that doctor was a catalyst to a life-altering event. His chiropractor, Dr. Brad Glowaki of Champion Chiropractic, quickly addressed the

crucial to quality of life as you age and will help you eliminate and compensate properly for various injuries.

12. USING THE WRONG EQUIPMENT

There have been so many advances in fitness equipment that can be customized to your body, it hurts me to see people using outdated equipment that doesn't adapt to their body and puts unnecessary strain on spinal joints, knees, ankles, hips, wrists, shoulders, and elbows. As you age in years, paying attention to these details becomes much more important.

Fitness equipment has made incredible strides over the last five years. It adjusts to your body shape and body size, as well as to the length of your limbs and your fitness goals.

structural misalignments from the fall, and moved him out of pain. Corrections of long-standing problems were then reversed, and Toby noticed a dramatic increase in his overall health and complete functionality of his body. His chiropractic adjustments provided such excellent results, the restaurateur canceled the surgery!

With renewed hope, and his passion for health restored, Toby's chiropractor recommended the help of a personal trainer to work on the strength that Toby had lost from extensive inactivity. Working with great intensity, Toby exceeded his youthful surfing days and easily lost the weight. He then saw the need to increase his endurance after having a second child. He chose a motivating goal of completing a half marathon and continued working with his two health professionals to achieve maximum success.

Today Mr. Reece routinely surfs big waves in Indonesia that far exceed the challenges of his youth. He has no pain, and now enjoys two successful sushi restaurants in California called Mahe, with a third opening soon. This local hero is celebrated within two separate beach communities for his philanthropic donations to the elementary schools. Each year he heads an educational campaign at each of his restaurants to donate funds in excess of $50,000. Toby has truly modeled his life after The 100 Year Lifestyle and he has many supporters expecting him to be surfing for that birthday as well!

Unfortunately, many fitness centers have not upgraded their equipment in years. Working out on the wrong equipment can be detrimental to your health. Functional training using pulley systems and free motion technology is an excellent type of equipment that can work for your entire body. You will see that a lot of the exercises we recommend take this into account, because they strengthen your core and your body at the same time. They also adapt to your size and customize to your shape. This adaptive mechanism becomes more important as you age, especially if you have had previous injuries that have reduced or altered the normal range of motion of your shoulders, knees, hips, and spine. Adaptive technologies can prevent injuries from happening by avoiding improper body mechanics that can result from using fixed motion equipment. It is also important to vary the equipment that you use in addition to using it properly. Always use equipment that fits your body.

A few years ago I got into a routine where I was using a standard elliptical cross trainer for all of my endurance training. About three months into this routine I went out for a run and pulled my calf muscle. It took a few weeks of rest, adjustments, and stretching to get my calf to heal. During this time period, for endurance training, I switched to the stationary bike and as soon as I was able to, I got back on the elliptical. Four weeks later, the other calf muscle went. What I realized was that using the same elliptical over and over again exercised my calf muscles within a very fixed range of motion. When I went to use those muscles outside that fixed range it put an unnecessary strain on them, causing them to pull. To solve this problem I did two things: I began stretching those muscles more regularly and I began varying my endurance training.

Precor, the company who originally launched the elliptical many years ago, just came out with a new elliptical that meets the adaptation qualities that we're talking about here. Their AMT or Adaptive Motion Technology elliptical can act as a stair climber, a treadmill, and an elliptical, and you can vary this style of endurance training without ever leaving the machine or pushing a button. The AMT is the wave of the future for endurance training as well as for strength training. Equipment that adapts to your body is best for maximizing function and longevity.

13. USING EQUIPMENT IMPROPERLY

The first line in the first chapter of *The 100 Year Lifestyle* says: "Tell me something I don't know." If you have ever had somebody tell you that it would be good for you to lose weight, change eating styles, or get your ESS in shape and you have ever found yourself saying the words "I know," it may be time for you to know things, well, differently.

I was recently having a conversation with a friend of mine who happens to be a doctor. While he exercises regularly, fitness is not his specialty and he was asking me about some of the different exercises in The 100 Year Lifestyle Workout. When I described the functional training using pulleys for strength training, he said that he had seen people at the gym using those techniques but he thought they were "cheating" because they were using their entire body instead of just isolating those specific muscles. This was an interesting perspective because many people use equipment improperly and cheat by trying to force extra reps and putting their body into poor posture on equipment that is designed to keep your body in a fixed position. This is using the equipment improperly.

When you use fixed equipment it stabilizes and isolates specific muscles. This is how the equipment should be used. Functional training equipment with pulleys is designed so that you can use your entire body and incorporate complementary muscles into your workout. These techniques will strengthen your core as well as your entire body by using muscles as they are used in real life. Knowing how to use the different pieces of technology and equipment available today will help you prevent injuries and get more out of your fitness time. Getting a personal trainer to show you how to use the different equipment available in your gym can add versatility to your workouts, maximize your results, and minimize your chance of injury.

14. NO ACCURATE BASELINE STARTING POINT OR SYSTEM OF MONITORING

It is important to know where you are starting from if you want to get where you are going. Just like a GPS system needs your current location as well as your destination, so does your fitness

plan. Many people get started with their workouts and become frustrated because they don't feel like they are making progress. They look at the scale and see that they lost five pounds in the first two weeks, but in the second two weeks they haven't lost any. This can be frustrating; however, if you are lifting weights and increasing your muscle mass, your weight may not change but your percentage of body fat may go down. Your percentage of lean muscle mass may go up. If you are not aware of your starting points, and you do not monitor your progress, you can cause yourself some unnecessary frustration. In the following chapter you will get an assessment that gives you an accurate baseline as well as a way to monitor your progress. You can record these numbers by yourself, with a partner, or with a personal trainer. Either way, start measuring and start working out.

15. UNCLEAR GOALS OR VISION FOR YOUR NEW BODY AND HEALTH

Have specific fitness goals. When you are unclear about what you want your body to look like, you won't be able to measure your accomplishments and success will be harder to define. The beauty of The 100 Year Lifestyle Workout is that you can shape your body any way you want to through the lifestyle choices that you make. Do you want a leaner waist that measures thirty-two or thirty-four inches? Do you want to fit into a size four, six, eight? It is important to visualize your goals. Do you want more tone in your arms, back, or chest? Do you want to strengthen your legs or your spine? What do you want your weight and percentage of body fat to be? Having clear targets will keep you focused on your goals. Having unclear targets may lead to you being on a roller coaster.

16. BEING INCONSISTENT WITH YOUR WORKOUTS

Consistency is what The 100 Year Lifestyle is all about. If fitness is a part of your lifestyle, then you will eliminate the "should I or shouldn't I" workout conversations that may be plaguing your progress. Being inconsistent will keep you on the weight gain, weight loss roller coaster. In *The 100 Year Lifestyle,* I discussed the difference between being crisis motivated and quality of life motivated when it comes to healthy lifestyle choices. If inconsistency is one of your pitfalls, then you are probably crisis motivated. You wait until your pants don't fit and then you begin working out again. Maybe you wait until you have a reaction to a certain food and then you begin to avoid it again. Maybe you wait until you have a backache and then you get your chiropractic adjustment. Inconsistency is a habit. Consistency is a lifestyle.

By now you are probably motivated and on your way to making fitness a part of your ideal 100 Year Lifestyle. Your fitness has become a priority and you know what not to do. The next chapter will give you the structure to begin measuring your baseline, your progress, and your results so that you make the most of your 100 Year Lifestyle Workout program.

CHAPTER THREE:

Measure Your Success: Simple Strategies for Tracking Fitness and Nutrition

Whether you are just beginning a fitness plan, trying to break through a plateau, or trying to break a record, you should measure your progress. This raises several questions: What should you measure? How do you measure? How often should you measure? I will answer these questions in this chapter.

If you are a new exerciser, over forty, and out of shape, get an examination by your cardiologist to make sure your heart is healthy, and by your chiropractor to make sure your spine is healthy enough for you to take on your fitness adventures. Now that this disclaimer is out of the way, call and make the appointment. Too many people postpone getting started on a fitness plan because they read this disclaimer everywhere and they never go ahead and make the appointment. So make the appointment. Your cardiologist will perform blood tests and measure your cholesterol levels, listen to your heart, and make sure that you are not one beat away from a heart attack. This is good information to know, and then he or she will recommend that you begin a fitness plan.

Your chiropractor will examine your spine for alignment, balance, and nerve pressure that can cause all types of health problems. If indicated, he or she will also perform a computerized spinal and/or x-ray examination to thoroughly evaluate the structure and function of your spine and nervous system. These tests give you insights that can improve your fitness plan, and can also discover underlying conditions in your spine that can limit your overall health and quality of life as you age, or lead to unnecessary injuries.

The challenge is that sometimes the first available appointment can be weeks or months away, and if the new exerciser doesn't start on a program, the appointment comes and the new exerciser has lost his or her motivation to get started. Don't let this happen to you. Call and make your appointment today. There are some exercises, such as power walking, that you can do to get rolling that are safe and healthy and that can help you immediately capitalize on your internal motivation.

MEASURING MADE SIMPLE

Many of us don't want to measure; we just want to start. We are not left brain or analytical in any way, shape, or form, and the thought of measuring becomes extremely overwhelming to us. Don't allow the fear of measuring to keep you from starting. Consider enlisting the help of a fitness professional. Starting with a personal trainer who can do the measuring for you can make the process simple and easy for you to do. Find an environment that you like in a gym or personal training studio and make an appointment. Measuring your starting point helps you monitor your progress and see your improvement.

We all know that people with the best bodies, or athletes who are in the best shape, measure. Bodybuilders measure the size of their muscles, their body fat, and the amount of calories they burn and consume in a day among other things. Sprinters measure how fast they run or swim. During their workouts, they consistently measure to see their progress and when they hit a plateau they change up their training to try and take themselves over the hump. Football players, depending on their position, measure how far they can throw, how quick they can run a forty-yard dash, or how much weight they can lift. Basketball players measure how high they can jump. Baseball players measure how fast they can throw the ball. Measuring is a part of every sport and the more serious you get about your fitness plan, the more you are going to want to measure. Don't let the thought of measuring overwhelm you and keep you from starting this program. Did I say that already? Great, if you have decided to start, you should also decide to measure.

Here are some ways to measure yourself from simple to more complex. The key is to get started on your plan and become more sophisticated as you learn more about being fit and healthy. Remember life-changing principle #2: Think progress, not perfection.

- Scale—measures your total body weight

- Tape measure—measures the size of your chest, waist, hips, muscles, and other body parts

- Pedometer—measures the number of steps you take

- Heart monitor—measures the number of heartbeats per minute and the number of calories you burn during your workouts. More sophisticated heart monitors can measure how much time you spend in your target heart rate zone and many other things as well.

- Body fat analyzer—measures the percentage of body fat you have

- Body composition analyzer—in addition to measuring your percentage of body fat, this can also measure the percentage of lean body mass, muscle, or water you have to determine if your body composition is balanced

- Basal metabolic rate—how many calories your body burns in a day at rest

- Calorie counter—measures the amount of

Maintain a healthy weight and body composition. Your body fat should be between 12 and 18 percent for men and between 14 and 22 percent for women.

calories you burn during your workouts and over the course of an entire day. There are online calorie counters where you can measure your calorie intake and the number of calories you burn and consume in a day. Try this at www.100yearlifestyle.com and also see the chapter on nutrition. There are arm bands that you can wear to get your personal calorie count exactly.

- Posture analysis—this measures your structure and whether or not your spine is balanced

- Bilateral scale—measures your weight balance on one side of your body compared to the other

- Electromyograph (EMG)—measures the electrical conductivity of the spinal nerves that supply your muscles. Can be done at many chiropractic offices.

- Electrointerstitial Scan (EIS)—measures the interstitial fluid for an overview of your body chemistry balance and composition.

- Electocardiograph (EKG)—measures the electrical conductivity in your heart.

- Blood tests—measure you on the inside and can be performed by your doctor. You can get your blood cholesterol levels, good and bad cholesterol, blood sugar levels, and a lot of additional information on how you are doing on the inside, as opposed to just seeing what is on the outside.

Your 100 Year Lifestyle Measurements

If you are ready to measure and go, and you want to skip all of the explanations, then there is a chart at the end of this chapter where you can just begin to fill in the numbers and get rolling. Go to www.100yearlifestyle.com and log into the online fitness personal trainer, or take the chart to your chiropractor, personal trainer, or cardiologist and let them help you fill in the blanks with the appropriate testing.

Congratulations on your motivation and your passion for jumping in full speed ahead. If you are more cautious about getting started but are ready to go, keep reading and I will give you some simpler ways to measure your progress and your success.

Easy Measuring for Beginners Who Insist on Starting by Themselves

I know that no matter what I say and what professional I recommend that you see, some of you will not seek the advice from your doctor or fitness professional and you will either get started on your own, or not start. If I just described you, then you should still get started, and you should still measure. These suggestions will make it easy for you.

First step on the scale and check your weight. Second look on the inside of your pants at the waist size—this will measure your waist. This is enough to get started. Now get moving.

The easiest things to measure when you start exercising are the Frequency, Intensity, and Duration of your workouts. If you are a beginner and you are getting started on your own without the help of a doctor or health care provider, you can measure the above in some very simple ways.

Measure your frequency by tracking how often you exercise. Is it once a day, five times a week, or three times a week? If you are new to fitness and feel overwhelmed by your body, how much weight you want to eliminate, and the fear of the unknown, then just get moving. Decide to go for a ten-minute walk every day. Your frequency here is seven days per week and at least you are measuring something. Your duration in this case would be ten minutes.

You can measure your intensity by buying a pedometer for less than $20 and counting the number of steps you take during your walk. You can increase your intensity by increasing the number of steps you take during your walk. Try increasing the number of steps you take by 10 percent after your first week. When you increase

ESS Story: Matt Beerman

I have always known that exercise and good eating habits are important. Knowing that and doing something about it are two very different things. From time to time I have made my health a priority, and over the years I had my moments where I'd been in really good shape and then not so good shape. I would get motivated to get back into shape occasionally because I was going on a cruise or I had to completely exhale in order to tie my shoes. But even after all that hard work, I would go right back into my old routine by slacking off on my diet and not going to the gym as often.

I decided to start the Gold's Gym Challenge. My thought process was really not any different—I wanted to get back into shape because summer was just around the corner and I wanted to look better in shorts—and by that I mean I wanted to get rid of my love handles. The Gold's Gym Challenge seemed like a good way to add some spice to this year's fitness break.

Shortly after joining the challenge it became apparent that things were different this time. I now had a daughter who, at the beginning of the challenge, was seven months old. I would think about how great it would be to coach her soccer team someday or play with her in the park, take her hiking or go for a bike ride together. All of which would be hard to do if I was only in shape for special occasions. It became quite

your intensity, your workouts will become more efficient; you will burn more calories, and your results will begin to increase. This is an easy way to measure and it is exciting when you begin to see your progress. If you have been consistent for two weeks, you can increase all three components of your beginning plan by bringing your duration to twenty minutes and increasing the number of steps you take per minute by monitoring your results on the pedometer.

To add strength to your program, add the Core Strength and Stability test in the Go Core Crazy chapter, and do the best you can with it. See how far you get with it and this will be what you measure.

After four weeks of beginning your Get Your ESS in Shape program, you will have more confidence in yourself because you will see results, and you can now begin to add the other elements of the ESS to your workout. Now is the

clear early on in the challenge that more would come of this than just looking better in shorts for the summer.

I believe it was Dr. Plasker's opening lecture that was really the eye opener for me. I am going to live until I'm at least 100 years old! Which means, I still have sixty years to go. My first thought was, why change my routine? I can still get into shape when I need to and the rest of the time be a couch potato. But actually, sixty or so up and down cycles didn't sound so exciting. Besides, those cycles seemed to keep getting harder and harder the older I got. It was definitely time for me to face the facts—I needed to get my ESS in shape and stay in shape if I wanted to live a quality life until 100.

The routine was a lot easier than I thought it would be. It also helped bring my wife and me together with a common goal and common timeframe. She and I went to the gym together and took turns motivating each other. We tried new things, like spinning classes. We went to the seminars and measurement sessions together, which really kept us involved in each other's progress. It helped me to stay motivated when I knew she was depending on me to get her to the gym and not take her to McDonald's for french fries.

After twelve weeks, I'd lost twenty-two pounds and reduced my body fat by 12 percent. I am looking forward to enjoying my 100 Year Lifestyle for decades.

time to visit the gym and start the beginner ESS training regimens in this book, or consult with a personal trainer and take some more detailed measurements. Just like your success has been motivating you so far, the more you measure the more success you will see and the more committed you will become. You will make measuring a part of your lifestyle.

MEASURING CALORIE INTAKE AND EXPENDITURE

A major challenge with getting in shape and managing your weight in our very busy high tech world is the invisibility of the slow and steady weight gain that eventually leads to you becoming overweight and obese. Think about this: Eating a mere ten extra calories per day above your daily needs results in one pound gained by the end of a year and thirty pounds of unintentional weight gain by the midpoint of your life span.

This is exactly what happened to me, and I know this is what has happened to many of you. Not knowing or seeing your weight gain occurring remains half the battle. If you become aware of your daily energy, calorie intake, and any imbalances that may be occurring, you will be able to gain control over your body and regulate your food intake and movement level to keep your ESS in shape. As you become aware of the amount of food and calories that you are taking in, you can adjust your lifestyle and manage your weight more successfully.

We all have access to large quantities of nutrient-dense, inexpensive food coupled with the innate tendency to eat whatever is on our plates. For many of us, we eat unconsciously. Becoming conscious and purposefully changing your behavior may be the only non-invasive way to consistently offset these forces. Being aware of the calories you consume and expend will help you effectively manage your weight and keep you on target toward reaching your goals. Monitoring your calories will also help you make decisions on whether to alter your food intake or increase your activity level to stay on track.

Understanding Calories and Weight Control

Weight control is ultimately determined by calories. Simply put, if you are in calorie balance, then you are burning the same number of calories that you are taking in; if you are in a calorie surplus, then you are consuming more calories than you are burning, which will cause you to gain weight. Finally, if you are in a calorie deficit, then you are burning more calories than you are consuming, which will result in weight loss.

If you truly want to control your weight, you need to know how many calories you require on a daily basis. This varies according to your age, height, weight, lean body mass, gender, and activity level. Human beings require a continuous source of energy to fuel our basal metabolic rate (BMR), physical activity, and the thermic effect of food (TEF). Your BMR accounts for the majority of your daily energy needs and includes maintenance of normal bodily functions such as breathing, circulation, and central nervous system activity. Various methods exist to measure your BMR accurately including direct and indirect calorimetry. Direct calorimetry measures the heat produced by your body in a closed chamber, while indirect calorimetry uses the amount of oxygen taken in and the carbon dioxide released. These methods are expensive and impractical for most people and instead, several prediction equations, most commonly Harris Benedict, are used to estimate your BMR. Once you determine your BMR, you will know how to adjust your lifestyle to support your fitness and weight management goals.

Physical activity makes up approximately 20 percent of your energy expenditure, and your calorie requirements vary according to the amount of activity you do. The digestion and absorption of food also requires energy and accounts for approximately 10 percent of daily energy expenditure. The rest of your innate bodily functions, such as breathing, also require energy, and all these components determine the number of calories you require on a daily basis

To calculate your basal metabolic rate, visit www.100yearlifestyle.com to sign up for the free fourteen-day trial.

for your weight to remain stable. Once you have an estimation of your daily requirements, you can add calories or subtract them depending on what you want to achieve. Without this knowledge you are playing a guessing game that can be very frustrating and keep you on the roller coaster ride that you are trying to get off.

Tracking Calories Improves Success

The longest and most comprehensive scientific study comparing different weight loss diets has confirmed that weight loss occurs when calories are reduced, regardless of the type of diet. Research has also demonstrated that those who consistently track what they eat lose more weight and are more successful at keeping the weight off. The act of writing down the items and quantities you habitually consume increases your awareness of your eating habits, which is important if you want to change the behaviors that lead to excessive calorie intake.

If you are like most people, you may be unaware of the calorie content of the items you frequently consume. One study revealed that participants underestimated a large meal by up to one thousand calories. By consuming an additional one thousand calories (which equates to a coffee drink and a muffin) once a week without making up for it with more activity, you would experience a fifteen-pound weight gain after one year. Through the process of tracking your calories, you will gain the knowledge of calorie intake, portion sizes, and alternative, healthier choices—all essential for long-term weight control, health, and longevity.

Online Food Logging is Easy, and Can Be Done from Anywhere

Now you can easily track your calories online. Food logging, which is an important element of your 100 percent conscious day and regaining control over your lifestyle, has traditionally been done through a paper journal. Unfortunately, the information about the foods you eat is not always readily available. Online trackers have gained tremendous popularity recently, and technology is now providing Internet-based solutions that enable people to obtain services they would not normally seek due to cost, location, or time constraints.

Online programs can also provide social support and personalized feedback while allowing you to remain anonymous, thus avoiding any potential embarrassment that beginners may have with face-to-face programs. Indeed, Internet weight loss and weight management programs that incorporate behavioral principles have been shown to improve weight loss and help people reach their goals.

Through www.100yearlifestyle.com, powered by dotFIT, you can get started with your calorie tracking right away as well as create customized meal plans and much more to help you reach your goals.

Your Personal Trainer Online

The 100 Year Lifestyle nutrition and exercise program, powered by dotFIT, addresses all of the important issues we've discussed by providing you with greater awareness about your daily energy and calorie balance, including daily and weekly predicted weight loss or gain when you log your food and activity levels. It provides daily calorie intake and burn targets based on your personal goals and parameters, including your BMR. To increase awareness of environmental influences on food intake and your current eating habits, it includes an easy-to-use optional food logging application with an

The 5 Eats of a Healthy 100 Year Lifestyle Are . . .

1. Eat a healthy breakfast.

2. Eat a high-fiber diet rich with live (not processed) foods.

3. Eat healthy snacks.

4. Eat slowly.

5. Eat with others.

extensive CalorieKing food database along with various educational tools, tips, articles, and videos. Regardless of whether you log your food, after each weekly weigh-in you receive individualized feedback based on weight changes, and it offers specific suggestions as needed. It also provides progress charts, reports, and daily journals as they have also been shown to improve weight loss outcomes.

To increase your success and adherence to your plan, there are various options for coaching—either by e-mail, phone, or in person with a fitness professional. Extensive social support is provided with Web chats, message boards, and videos. These features give you the information you need to self-regulate your behavior and also include strategies for how to make any needed adjustments to your plan. There are other elements of the 100 Year Lifestyle dotFit Me Program that include:

- Numerous menus designed by registered dietitians—including athletic performance, vegetarian, specialty (Mediterranean diet, lactose intolerant, 40/30/30), and lifestyle menus (healthy fast food, night out). Sample seven-day plans are provided separately.

- A vast library of articles, videos, and frequently asked questions on weight loss, health, exercise, nutrition, performance, women's health, senior health, and youth topics

- Personalized dietary support recommendations based on a health screening and your goals

- Walking and exercise programs designed by the National Academy of Sports Medicine. Programs are based on the goal, desired workout frequency, duration, and type of equipment available and video demos are included for each exercise

- Option to add a body monitoring device to track calories burned, steps, and activity

Go to 100yearlifestyle.com and start playing around with this incredible tool right now.

The 100 Year Lifestyle dotFIT Me program provides a comprehensive twenty-first century solution that addresses the challenges of weight control in today's environment. This program will absolutely help you get and keep your ESS in shape. It is fun, informative, and you can log into your personal account from any location so it can help you stay on track when you are traveling. As new methods and tools emerge with science and technology, we are committed to providing you these fresh solutions and partnering with those who are passionate and committed to helping others succeed through The 100 Year Lifestyle.

EMPTY CALORIES (ECs) VS. QUALITY CALORIES (QCs)

When you are faced with food choices, it is important to consider the *type* of calories that you are consuming. Ask yourself are these ECs or empty calories, or are they QCs, quality calories? Unfortunately for many people their diet consists of an excessive amount of calories that are also ECs. When this happens not only will you gain weight, but you will become deficient in essential nutrients that your body needs in order to be healthy. What makes an EC an EC is that it is devoid of vitamins, minerals, antioxidants, electrolytes, or fiber. ECs include foods such as cookies, cakes, ice cream, white breads, and white pastas that provide your body with calories, but have no significant nutritional content. When your diet is filled with empty calories, they will not satisfy your hunger because, while your belly may be full, your cells will crave the nutrients. This creates a vicious cycle that explains why people with high EC intake become and stay obese.

QCs on the other hand, or quality calories, come from foods that are live, lean, and healthy. These include fresh fruits and vegetables, lean meats and proteins, as well as 100 percent whole grains. QCs not only give you calories, but they also give you nutrition, which your body needs to function well and at a high level.

100 Year Lifestyle Foods

Examples of ECs, Empty Calories
Bagels
Beer
Breads made with white flour
Brownies
Cake
Candy
Cereals, sugary
Cinnamon rolls
Cookies
Croissants
Danish
Doughnuts
French fries
Pancakes, made with white flour
Soft drinks

Examples of QCs, Quality Calories
Apples
Asparagus
Avocados
Brown rice
Cruciferous vegetables, such as broccoli
    and brussels sprouts
Edamame
Eggplant
Whole wheat pasta with tomato sauce and/
    or vegetables
Peaches
Sweet potatoes, baked

100 Year Lifestyle Foods
Raw walnuts, Raw almonds, Raw cashews
Beans and other legumes
Spinach and other green vegetables
Oatmeal
Turkey and other lean meats (lean steak,
    chicken, fish)
Extra virgin olive oil
Whole-grain breads and cereals
Organic raspberries
Organic blueberries
Organic strawberries

For great, healthy recipes filled with lots of QCs, visit www.100yearlifestyle.com.

On page 50 you will find a short list of ECs and QCs, and a more extensive one can be found at www.100yearlifestyle.com.

When you adjust your calories to match your metabolism, you may experience some bouts with hunger pangs. If you are used to eating more calories than your body needs and you cut back on your calorie intake, your body may send you a reminder that you need to eat more through hunger pangs. Take control of your mind and your pangs. Tracking your calories can really help you here because you will know that you are not really hungry and your body does not really need more food; you have just been trained to overeat. Changing your eating habits and adjusting your lifestyle to your metabolism will eventually cause your hunger pangs to disappear. In fact, you may find yourself going in completely the opposite direction, feeling disgusted when you feel stuffed. Finding the balance here is important, which is why knowing your BMR and counting your calories play such a crucial role in your long-term success.

If you grow your own food, or you shop completely organic and your diet is very clean, you may not need to supplement. However, if you live in the twenty-first century in an industrial society, then it probably makes sense for you to add some type of supplementation to your diet. Your supplements should be derived from foods and packaged without fillers and preservatives. They should be filled with a high concentration of B vitamins, antioxidants, and omega-3 fatty acids. At the time of this writing, we are searching for the top supplements that we believe will support your optimum health with this exercise program, and you can find this information on www.100yearlifestyle.com.

MEASURING ENDURANCE

During your heart examination with your doctor, he or she will measure your heart health. To measure your endurance during your workouts, you will use a heart monitor. The workouts that follow in the next section give you a baseline of

---

Calculating Your Target Heart Rate Training Range

Start by calculating your Maximal Heart Rate (MHR). Multiply your MHR by upper and lower percentages to calculate your Target Heart Rate (THR) range.

1. Calculate your approximate Maximal Heart Rate (MHR) by subtracting your age from 220.
   Example: 220 – 45 (age) = 175 (MHR of a forty-five-year-old)

2. Then to calculate your Target Heart Rate (THR) range, multiply the MHR by 60 percent and 90 percent.

Example: 175 x .60 = 105   175 x .90 = 158

Therefore the THR range for a forty-five-year-old is between 105 and 158 beats per minute.

exercises that you can start with, and you should wear a heart monitor at all times when you work out. Follow the plan and record the Frequency, Intensity, and Duration of your workouts. Track your intensity by measuring the number of calories that you burn during your workouts. As your intensity increases, you will also find that your endurance increases. Set goals as to the number of calories that you want to burn during your workouts. You will see that as time goes on, your workouts get easier and your calorie burn goes up. This is a great way to measure your progress. Continue to adjust your goals to your progress so that you break through plateaus and see constant improvement in your ESS.

As your Beginner workouts get easier, try the Intermediate and then the Advanced workouts. Vary the intensity as your stamina increases and you will increase your endurance. You will find that if you are taking in enough quality calories to offset your energy burn, your endurance will skyrocket and your energy level will soar. If you find that your energy level gets low, it may be that you need to consume more quality calories to ensure the proper energy balance that you need to stay sharp, focused, and healthy. You may find that you need to time your meals and snacks differently. This is where The 100 Year Lifestyle dotFIT Me program can also be helpful by tracking your calorie intake.

Varying your intensity can improve your results. University of Alberta researchers reported in September that a group of healthy people who wore pedometers and made an effort to take an extra five thousand steps a day (about fifty minutes of walking) showed no improvement in their physical fitness after six months. But another group that hit the gym only four days a week for forty minutes of moderately intense workouts (visualize walking as fast as you can without actually running) significantly increased their endurance levels. In essence, the greater your intensity, the more efficient your workouts. A study published in the September *Journal of Physiology* compared two groups of cyclers who engaged in six exercise sessions over two weeks and found that those who did thirty-second sprints mixed with four-minute rest periods for thirty minutes had the same improvements as those who biked at a moderately intense pace for more than ninety minutes. According to the *Journal of Physiology*, "All-out sprints call every muscle cell into action, while traditional endurance workouts allow some cells to sit there dormant."

Vary your intensity and you will improve your results and also keep your body's adaptation mechanism fooled, which will help you break through plateaus.

MEASURING STRENGTH

As you begin the strength element of your workouts, you should start with a specific amount of weight that allows you to complete each set of the exercise you are doing with some extra effort required for your eighth to your twelfth repetitions. After a few weeks you will realize that the last few reps begin to get easier. If you want to bulk up, this is the time to increase the amount of weight you are using. If you want to stay lean and toned without bulking up, increase the number of repetitions that you do by 50 percent prior to adding more weight. Either way, this is a sure sign that your strength is improving.

Monitor your strength as your workouts improve over time through the amount of the weights that you use and the number of repetitions that you do. Some days will be easier than others and some days will be harder than others. Over time, however, you will find that your strength is increasing and this will bring with it a more toned body and a higher level of personal confidence that comes with being stronger. As you age, your commitment to maintaining your strength will give you the independence that you want and the ability to do more and experience more of what life has to offer.

MEASURING STRUCTURE

Measuring your overall spinal health will be done through the simple posture test that follows as well as your spinal examinations with your chiropractor. Measuring and maintaining good posture during your workouts will ensure that you maximize the quality of your workouts and your results, while also minimizing your risk of injury.

Proper posture during all of your exercises is extremely important. A computer scan of your spine or an x-ray can give you a lot of information about the underlying health of your spine and nervous system, whereas a general posture scan can give you an overview. You can do a simple self-posture test to determine if your spine is growing properly. To begin, stand in front of a mirror and close your eyes. Stand up as straight as you can. March in place for approximately ten steps and then open your eyes and answer the following questions:

- Look at your shoulders. Is one higher than the other?

- Look at your belt height. Is one side higher than the other?

- Look at the top of your ears. Is one higher than the other?

- Is your head hunched forward in front of your shoulders?

- Is your belly sticking forward and is there an excessive arch in your back?

Have your spouse, a friend, or your trainer take a picture of you from the back and from the side. Do you see any of the imbalances that were just mentioned above? These are signs that your structure is out of balance and when you work out, you should pay special attention to your posture.

The health of your spine and nervous system through proper alignment, chiropractic adjustments, and good posture is essential to quality of life as you age. Too many people are crisis motivated when it comes to caring for the lifeline of their bodies. Quality of life motivation is a much better option. Instead of being motivated by pain, be motivated by balance. Rather than letting fatigue motivate you, be motivated by healthy nerve supply and optimum energy.

I just returned from seeing one of my chiropractors at Healthquest Chiropractic in Marietta, Georgia. I have been traveling a lot and working on tight deadlines to complete this book. I was run down and I didn't even know it. My adjustment removed the pressure and energized my system. I don't know how people function without this care. They certainly are not functioning at 100 percent. Try it for yourself and see the difference that it makes in your life to have your spine and nerve system functioning to its full potential.

All three elements of the ESS—endurance, strength, and structure—are essential for quality of life as you age. The balance of these three will keep you functioning at a high level into your golden years. Giving your body the right fuel is the next important element of this plan. Turn the page and enjoy the lifestyle nutrition strategies to keep you lean, healthy, and energetic for a lifetime.

Personal Measurements

Starting — Bicep _____ Tricep _____ Subscapular _____ Suprailiac ____
Measurements — Weight _____ Body fat % _____ LBM _____ BFM _____
Body Composition — Neck _____ Chest _____ U Arm _____ F Arm _____
Measurements: — Waist _____ Hip _____ Thigh _____ Calf _____

6 Weeks — Bicep _____ Tricep _____ Subscapular _____ Suprailiac ____
Measurements — Weight _____ Body fat % _____ LBM _____ BFM _____
Body Composition — Neck _____ Chest _____ U Arm _____ F Arm _____
Measurements: — Waist _____ Hip _____ Thigh _____ Calf _____

12 Weeks — Bicep _____ Tricep _____ Subscapular _____ Suprailiac ____
Measurements — Weight _____ Body fat % _____ LBM _____ BFM _____
Body Composition — Neck _____ Chest _____ U Arm _____ F Arm _____
Measurements: — Waist _____ Hip _____ Thigh _____ Calf _____

6 Months — Bicep _____ Tricep _____ Subscapular _____ Suprailiac ____
Measurements — Weight _____ Body fat % _____ LBM _____ BFM _____
Body Composition — Neck _____ Chest _____ U Arm _____ F Arm _____
Measurements: — Waist _____ Hip _____ Thigh _____ Calf _____

Your changes — Weight _____ Body fat % _____ LBM _____ BFM _____

Your subscapular area is on your back at the base of your "wing" bones. Your suprailiac area is on your sides at the top of your pelvic bones. LBM and BFM stands for lean body mass and body fat mass. U Arm and F Arm are your upper arm and forearm.

Meal Tracking

In order to help you track your intake and workouts, we recommend that you keep a food diary during the first weeks of your journey towards getting your ESS in Shape. On this page, you can track your meals and snacks as well as your daily workout. Please make copies of this page to use in documenting your progress.

Date _____   M T W Th F Sa Su

Breakfast _____
Snack _____
Lunch _____
Snack _____
Dinner _____
Snack_____

Today's Workout
Endurance _____   Strength _____   Structure_____

Date _____   M T W Th F Sa Su

Breakfast _____
Snack _____
Lunch _____
Snack _____
Dinner _____
Snack_____

Today's Workout
Endurance _____   Strength _____   Structure_____

Date _____   M T W Th F Sa Su

Breakfast _____
Snack _____
Lunch _____
Snack _____
Dinner _____
Snack_____

Today's Workout
Endurance _____   Strength _____   Structure_____

Track your meals online at www.100yearlifestyle.com.

CHAPTER FOUR:

Eat Right: Nutrition and Meal Plans to Reach Your Goals

"The doctor of the future will give no medicine, but will interest his patients in the care of the human frame, in diet, and in the cause and prevention of disease."

—THOMAS EDISON

Fitness is a great word, especially if you like to have fun with acronyms. In order to be fit, you need to address the "NESS," Nutrition along with your Endurance, Strength, and Structure. We will examine nutrition in this chapter from a very practical perspective of healthy eating and managing your calories, in a way that is relevant and easy to implement in our modern day world.

When you visit www.100yearlifestyle.com and click on Get Your ESS in Shape, you will find many menu options on the 100 Year Lifestyle dotFIT Me program, and you can customize your meal plans. All menus were created by registered dietitians and are based on individual eating styles, preferences, and lifestyle. Below you will find a variety of sample menu options that are enjoyable to eat and will help you reach your goals depending on your size and BMR. I have listed 1,250-calorie menus that will result

in weight loss and improved health outcomes for many women and 2,000-calorie menus that will result in weight loss and better health for most men. Daily calories and foods should be adjusted according to your needs and preferred nutrient levels as well as activity levels. When you go to the Web site and put in your personal information and goals, the Web site will calculate a healthy calorie count for you. The target calories are listed for each meal so that any food or meal on the site can be substituted as long as the calories are followed. Calorie-free beverages such as water, or unsweetened tea and coffee, can be consumed as desired. You can also create menus for improving athletic performance or gaining muscle mass, in addition to losing weight. These menus will require additional calories so that you provide your body with the energy it needs to sustain you throughout the day and give you the body composition you are looking to achieve.

Standard Menu—1,258 calories

This is an ideal menu based on the Dietary Guidelines for Americans, published by the Department of Health and Human Services, and contains mostly whole grains, three to five servings of fruits and vegetables, and at least 25 grams of fiber.

Breakfast—Yogurt with cereal, fruit, and nuts, 335 calories

> 1 container (6 ounces) nonfat vanilla yogurt
> ½ cup fresh berries
> ⅓ cup bran cereal
> 1 ounce natural almonds (23 pieces)

Lunch—Soup, sandwich, and fruit, 438 calories

> 1 cup (8 ounces) low-sodium tomato soup
> 2 slices whole wheat bread
> 2 slices (1 ounce) lowfat cheddar cheese
> 1 medium orange

Dinner—Beef tacos and fruit, 395 calories

> 2 whole wheat low-carb tortillas
> 2 ounces cooked ground beef, 95% lean
> Lettuce, tomato, and onion as desired
> 2 tablespoons light sour cream
> 1 ounce avocado
> 1 cup diced melon

Dessert—Low calorie treat, 90 calories

> ½ cup lowfat, low sugar chocolate pudding

Nutrient breakdown: 50% carbohydrate, 22% protein, 28% fat, 3% saturated fat, 94 mg cholesterol, 44 g fiber, 1,817 mg sodium.

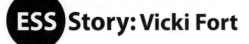

ESS Story: Vicki Fort

I am one of those people who has fought a lifelong battle with my weight. As a child I was always overweight, because I ate whatever looked good to me whether it was mealtime or not, whether I was really hungry or not. I have often joked that I was on a "See Food Diet." I'd see food and I'd eat it.

By the time I reached age fifty, I'd eaten my way to obesity, and I had terrible left leg pain all of the time. I was on medication for blood pressure, three asthma inhalers, a pill for my asthma, and cholesterol medication, which was causing other problems with body aches. I eventually had what turned out to be extensive back surgery, which included the removal of a cyst, a bone spur, and the fusion of two vertebrae.

I was good about exercising for the first year after surgery. I managed to pile up about three hundred miles while walking around town and on my treadmill. Then the pain returned, in my right leg this time, and I slipped back into my old mindset that I was too heavy to exercise and that I would start again as soon as I lost some of my weight. Of course, I gained back what little bit I had lost and then some.

My lack of activity and the return of the weight did little to help the pain that I was feeling. I was not able to stand or walk for more than five minutes at a time without feeling a sharp, stabbing pain and terrible cramps—not a good thing when you like teaching and going to car shows and craft fairs. As the pain increased my patience with my students and my desire to go places with my husband and grandchildren decreased. During this time, I faithfully saw my chiropractor, Dr. Donna Stackpool in Lake Geneva, Wisconsin, seeking relief from the pain. Try as I might, my weight was fighting every step of the way.

The turning point for me finally came when a doctor sat me down, looked me straight in the eye, and said: "Vicki, you are fat and if you don't get rid of the weight, you could be in a wheelchair within the next five years and you will need to have another back surgery. I want you to lose at least 110 pounds." Wow!! What a wake-up call that was!

Yes, I had been told that I needed to lose weight before, but I had never had someone put it to me so bluntly. She also told me the name of the eating plan that she wanted me to be on and that she wanted me to start taking a water aerobics class immediately.

The diet part was easy. I'd done that many times before. The exercise was another story altogether. Thankfully, a friend of mine offered to sign up for the aerobics class with me. She knows me well enough to know that I would be more likely to go to class if I knew that someone else was depending on me to go to class with them. After two classes, I was addicted. I couldn't wait until Wednesday night so that I could go to my aerobics class.

With a lot of hard work and determination the weight started to fall off. I felt so much better both physically and mentally, because I was doing something that I knew was good for me and I was in complete control. For the first time in my long career as a dieter, I didn't feel deprived when I couldn't have all of that wonderful pasta and all of the fattening candy and yummy desserts. I really wanted to be thinner and I had finally found a way to do it.

Of course, the pain didn't disappear as quickly as the weight did. I still had doctors who felt that I would need immediate surgery if I ever hoped to get rid of my pain. Thank goodness I discussed this with my chiropractor, and she agreed with me that more weight loss could very well give me the same results and that it would be more likely to be a lasting result.

Now twenty-two months later, I am ninety pounds lighter. My daily blood pressure medication has been reduced from two pills to one pill, my asthma is now truly under control, with just one pill and two inhalers when I need them, I am able to walk for hours without being in pain, and I am working to get rid of my cholesterol medication.

My weight loss has slowed, but I haven't gained very much of it back. I still feel great and I have more energy now than I ever remember having. I get a great joy out of the little reminders of where I used to be: my "fat pants" that fall off of me when I let go of them, a belt that didn't fit me two years ago and is now six inches too big, and the very best, being able to offer my sweater to someone who needs it and knowing that it won't be way too big on them.

Healthy Fast Food—1,256 calories

Use this menu on days when you're too busy to prepare or eat meals at home. It provides a lunch and dinner from healthy fast foods and remaining meals from dotFIT foods. Choose your favorite item(s) for any meal that closely matches the target calories.

Breakfast—Favorite dotFIT food, 330 calories

> 1 breakfast bar
> 1 large apple

Lunch—Favorite restaurant meal, 394 calories

> Subway 6-inch oven roasted turkey sandwich on wheat bread, light condiments
> 1 small banana

Dinner—Favorite restaurant meal, 532 calories

> McDonald's Asian salad with grilled chicken
> 1 package lowfat sesame ginger dressing
> 1 Fruit 'n' Yogurt Parfait with granola

Nutrient breakdown: 61% carbohydrate, 22% protein, 17% fat, 4% saturated fat, 100 mg cholesterol, 21 g fiber.

Night Out Menu—1,247 calories

This menu is designed for the days when you have a planned social occasion or dinner at a restaurant. It provides approximately one-third of your calories from dotFIT foods and the remaining calories are reserved for your night out.

Breakfast—dotFIT item and fruit, 275 calories

   1 breakfast bar/shake/protein stick
   1 small apple

Lunch—dotFIT item, 190 calories

   1 protein stick/bar/dessert

Dinner—Night out meal, 782 calories

   1 bowl P.F. Chang's wonton soup
   ½ dish P.F. Chang's garlic noodles
   ½ dish P.F. Chang's almond cashew chicken

Nutrient breakdown: 49% carbohydrate, 25% protein, 26% fat, 6% saturated fat, 10 mg cholesterol, 9 g fiber.

Athletic Performance Menu—1,297 calories

This menu has the ideal amount and ratios of protein, carbohydrates, and fat for individuals who participate in sport(s) or exercise regularly.

Breakfast—Morning meal, 367 calories
Eat this snack as soon as you wake up.

> ¾ cup Wheaties
> 1 cup skim milk
> 1 extra small banana

Lunch—Pre-training meal, 342 calories
Eat this meal 2½ to 3 hours before activity.

> 1 (2-ounce) pita bread
> 2 ounces oven roasted turkey meat, lean (3–4 slices depending on thickness)
> 1 slice (1 ounce) lowfat Swiss cheese
> Mustard as desired
> 1 medium orange
> Water/calorie-free beverage (16–24 ounces)

Pre-training Snack—110 calories
Eat this snack 10–40 minutes before workouts to maximize energy stores.

> Water as needed
> ½ breakfast bar

Post-training Snack—110 calories
Eat or drink this snack immediately after workouts to refill energy stores and enhance recovery.

> 1 cup (8 ounces) water
> ½ breakfast bar

Dinner—368 calories
Eat this meal within 1½ hours after your workout.

> 1 cup whole wheat spaghetti, cooked
> 2 ounces cooked ground beef, 90% lean
> ½ cup (4 ounces) marinara sauce
> Optional: 1 dotFIT Active Multivitamin
> Water as needed

Nutrient Breakdown: 63% carbohydrate, 23% protein, 14% fat, 4% saturated fat, 71 mg cholesterol, 19 g fiber, 2,056 mg sodium.

Vegetarian Menu—1,250 calories

This menu is designed for individuals who do not eat beef, chicken, or fish. Protein is provided from dairy, eggs, soy products, beans, and nuts. You may replace any of these items with the items of your choice.

Breakfast—279 calories

> 2 whole wheat lowfat waffles
> ½ cup mixed berries
> ½ cup (4 ounces) lowfat 2% cottage cheese

Lunch—411 calories

> 1 package (10 ounces) Amy's Enchilada and Black Bean vegetarian meal, frozen
> 1 small pear

Snack—195 calories

> 1 medium banana
> 1 tablespoon natural creamy peanut butter

Dinner—365 calories

> ½ cup cooked brown rice
> 4 ounces firm Nigari tofu
> 2 cups Chinese-style vegetables, frozen
> 2 tablespoons teriyaki marinade and sauce

Nutrient Breakdown: 59% carbohydrates, 19% protein, 22% fat, 5% saturated fat, 9 mg cholesterol, 31 g fiber, 2,096 mg sodium.

Heart Healthy Menu—1,260 calories

Based on the Mediterranean diet that emphasizes healthy fats, fish, whole grains, fruits, and vegetables.

Breakfast—413 calories

> 2 whole wheat waffles
> 1 tablespoon maple syrup
> 1 cup sliced strawberries
> 1 container plain yogurt, fat-free

Lunch—372 calories

> ⅛ crust whole wheat pizza dough
> 4 ounces pizza sauce
> 1 ounce mozzarella cheese (part skim)
> Mushrooms, peppers. onion, squash as desired
> 1 cup red or green grapes

Dinner—475 calories

> 4 ounces salmon, baked
> ½ cup cooked brown rice
> 1 cup cooked broccoli
> 1 teaspoon olive oil

Nutrient Breakdown: 52% carbohydrate, 20% protein, 28% fat, 6% saturated fat, 94 mg cholesterol, 23 g fiber, 1,548 mg sodium.

Standard Menu – 2,001 Calories

This is an ideal menu based on the Dietary Guidelines for Americans and contains mostly whole grains, at least five servings of fruits and vegetables, and 25 grams of fiber.

Breakfast—563 calories

> 1 cup Shredded Wheat cereal
> 1 tablespoon dried berries/raisins
> 1 cup skim milk
> 1 slice whole wheat toast
> 1 tablespoon whipped butter
> 1 teaspoon jam
> 1 medium banana

Lunch—596 calories

> 2 slices rye bread
> 4 ounces albacore tuna in water (drained)
> 1 tablespoon mayonnaise
> Lettuce, tomato, celery, and onion, as desired
> 1 medium pear
> 1 cup skim milk

Snack—236 calories

> 1 ounce almonds (22 each)
> 1 medium apple

Dinner—606 calories

> 5 ounces roasted chicken (breast only)
> 1 large (6.3-ounce) baked sweet potato
> 1 tablespoon whipped butter
> 2 cups romaine lettuce mix
> 1 tablespoon low-calorie balsamic vinaigrette
> 1 100% whole wheat dinner roll

Nutrient Breakdown: 42% carbohydrate, 32% protein, 26% fat, 7% saturated fat, 496 mg cholesterol, 25 g fiber.

Healthy Fast Food – 2,022 Calories

Use this menu on days when you're too busy to prepare or eat meals at home. It provides a lunch and dinner from healthy fast foods and remaining meals from dotFIT foods. Choose your favorite item(s) for any meal which closely matches the target calories.

Meal 1—Favorite dotFIT food and fruit, 292 calories

    1 dotFIT breakfast bar
    1 medium apple

Meal 2—Restaurant meal, 595 calories

    Subway footlong turkey breast sandwich
    1 package Subway apple slices

Meal 3—Favorite dotFIT food and fruit, 295 calories

    1 dotFIT protein stick
    1 medium banana

Meal 4—Restaurant meal, 840 calories

    1 McDonald's Grilled Chicken Sandwich
    1 McDonald's Southwest Salad with Grilled Chicken
    1 package McDonald's Southwest Dressing

Nutrient Breakdown: 56% carbohydrate, 24% protein, 20% fat, 6% saturated fat, 220 mg cholesterol, 23 g fiber, 4,833 mg sodium.

These menus are a great starting point to get you on track toward reaching your goals. If you haven't been to www.100yearlifestyle.com yet, now is a great time to start. When you log in, you will have access to all types of menu suggestions at your desired calorie level to help you lose weight, gain muscle, get in shape, improve the health of your heart, lower your blood sugar, and much more. There are additional educational articles that you can learn from and if you need to, you can even ask a coach to help you. Try the dotFIT supplements and food products. They are delicious and nutritious and can be an excellent part of your overall fitness plan.

If you want to get great results, it is not enough to read this book. You must take action. Go online now and then go on to the next chapter, which will give you the ESS sequences that will tighten you up and get you in the best shape of your life.

CHAPTER FIVE

Get Your ESS in Shape: ESS Sequences for the Beginner, Intermediate, and Advanced Exerciser

"Look well to the spine for the cause of disease."

—HIPPOCRATES

If you want to stay active and healthy as you age, you must address all three components of the ESS. Why is the balance of Endurance, Strength, and Structure important as you age? The E, as in Endurance Training, means cardiovascular exercise. Endurance Training will help you:

- lose weight

- burn fat

- gain the stamina needed to endure the challenges of everyday life while also preparing you for the marathon of your extended life span

> **ESS training is essential for quality of life as you age.**
>
> **E** = Endurance
>
> **S** = Strength
>
> **S** = Structure
>
> Lose weight, look great, and stand straight.

- reduce the effects of stress on your body

- help keep your heart healthy

Endurance training includes:

- running, walking, or hiking

- swimming

- bike riding, whether stationary, on the road, or in the mountains

- elliptical machines

- fitness classes including Pilates and Yoga

- any other type of activity that raises your heart rate

Endurance training combined with good nutrition will help keep your heart healthy and your arteries clear for eighty, ninety, 100 years and beyond. Endurance training by itself will give you a smaller version of yourself with basically the same shape. If you are shaped like a pear, you will become a smaller pear. If you are shaped like an apple, you will become a smaller apple.

If you are a man with the perfect V shape or a woman with the perfect hourglass shape, you will be a smaller version of your current shape if you just do endurance training by itself.

The first "S" in ESS stands for Strength training. Strength training will:

- build muscle and keep your muscles toned

- keep your body lean

- help you to look great in a bathing suit or your boxers whether you are in your early twenties or near the century mark

- raise your lean body mass, which will help to increase your metabolism so that you naturally burn more calories (Some people have the ability to eat whatever they want without gaining weight because they are blessed with a naturally high metabolism. Strength training will add mass to your muscles and help your body burn more calories than if you were loose and flabby.)

- build and tone muscles almost immediately

- improve your strength

- improve your immune system

- reduce the effects of stress on your body

- reduce your percentage of body fat

- strengthen your bones

- give you more energy

- Strength training may raise your body weight. Since muscle weighs more than

fat, don't become alarmed if you feel better and look better but the number on the scale goes up slightly. Check your body composition for your percentage of body fat and make sure you are on track to reach your goals.

Strength training includes:
- weight training (barbells, dumbbells, or machines)
- pushups or pullups or any other type of exercise where you are adding resistance
- Pilates, Yoga, and many Les Mills group fitness classes that use weights

The final "S" in ESS stands for structure training. Structure training includes:

- stretching and flexibility

- good posture during all of your exercise

- developing a strong core, which includes your abdominal muscles, your hip flexors and extensors, and your lower back muscles

Structure training will help you:

- stand up straight

- improve your balance

- maintain or increase your flexibility regardless of how old you are

- keep the muscles around your spine strong and flexible

Good posture is important no matter what type of exercise you do—whether it's endurance training, sitting on a bike or lifting even the mildest of weights. In fact, having a healthy structure will very often determine the level of endurance and strength training that you can achieve.

Your ESS Program will help you to decrease your body fat and increase the tone of your muscles. Since muscle burns more calories than fat, by implementing the 100 Year Lifestyle Workout, you can raise your basal metabolic rate so that your body burns more calories even when it is resting.

Health problems can occur when your ESS is out of balance. As you will see, this can be very detrimental to your health.

ENDURANCE WITHOUT STRENGTH AND STRUCTURE

Several years ago I took care of a marathon runner who was addicted to road racing. By the time he came to my chiropractic practice, he had run somewhere in the neighborhood of thirty marathons. He consistently ran between fifty and seventy-five miles per week and you could really see this excessive endurance training taking its toll on his body—because he was not also taking care of his strength and his structure. His lean body mass was very high—he had almost no body fat. His problem: He didn't do any strength training and his spine was a mess. His upper body was becoming extremely weak and he would fatigue easily when he was required to use it.

I remember when he came in for one of his adjustments with his family. His young child had to be lifted up and down several times, and I noticed how he huffed and puffed and became frustrated by his lack of strength. At forty-five years old this poor determined runner was running himself and his spine into unnecessary aging. The spacing between the bones in his lower neck, between his fifth and sixth cervical vertebrae, was equivalent to someone in their seventies or eighties. The same was true with the spacing in the bottom bones of his lower back. When he looked at his x-rays, he asked me "is this deterioration because of my age?" I said, "No, it's because your structure is out of balance and your spine is wearing out unevenly."

Strength training is important for quality of life as you age. Have you ever seen an older person struggle to get out of a chair? Many of the activities that we take for granted when we are younger, like pulling ourselves out of bed, getting up from a chair, lifting up children or grandchildren, moving a box, or walking up the stairs, all require strength. When you neglect your strength, you run the risk of compromising your independence as you age, and if you wait until you lose your strength to make it a priority, it takes a lot longer to get it back.

Endurance training is important to ensure a healthy heart and cardiovascular system, but if you are lacking strength you will find yourself out of balance with your ESS, and it will affect your ability to maintain high levels of activity as you age. Proper alignment of your spine is critical for healthy aging. If you were to look at someone from behind and examine his or her posture you would see that his or her ears, shoulders, and hips were level with a healthy spine. When you look at someone from the side, if he or she is healthy, you should not see any signs of hunchback, swayback, or a forward leaning of the head. You should see a balanced positioning of the hips, shoulders, and ears. When the spine becomes misaligned and the biomechanics of the individual segments of the spine become distorted, it can lead to uneven deterioration of the structure and the bones, while also causing deterioration of the nerves. This can not only weaken your muscles, but it can also affect the function of your vital organs as well.

Good structure keeps you aligned. Think about this: If the tires on your car are out of alignment and you leave the car parked in the driveway, will it matter that the tires are out of balance? Of course it won't. If you want to drive the car and you want to drive it faster and longer, then the alignment absolutely matters. When you drive a car with misaligned tires, you will feel a little pull to one side or the other. After a while, you'll notice that your gas mileage begins to go down because it requires more energy to drive. Additionally, as time goes on you will wear out the front end and the tires, and if you ignore the signals long enough you will be headed for a blowout. The same is true for your body when you do endurance training without strength and without good structural alignment and balance. At first, you may begin to fatigue a little quicker than normal. You'll start repeatedly pulling muscles with no explanation until

eventually you have a complete blowout. This doesn't have to happen to you. If you take care of your structure, you'll help maintain your alignment—just like a mechanic would do with your car. It's no wonder many major sports teams, top athletes and entertainers use a chiropractor to ensure their high-priced athletes function at the top of their game.

STRENGTH WITHOUT ENDURANCE AND STRUCTURE

Strength training, as we have discussed, is important for quality of life as you age. By itself, however, without endurance and structure training, it is not enough. One of my patients was a professional wrestler in the WWE. This very kind and fun man was huge in his physical appearance and packed an enormous amount of strength into his frame, but his constant neglect of his endurance and structure was limiting him. His overall health, along with his effectiveness in the ring, was impacted by the fact that he only paid attention to strength.

One day he came in for his adjustment and was in a particularly good mood. I was feeling a little frisky and in good fun I poked him in the chest and assumed a wrestler's position remembering my high school glory days. Before I could blink an eye he scooped me up and held me up in the air over his shoulders as if he was ready to give me the body slam of my life. Before he dropped me on my head I looked down on him and said, "please put me down and remember I am about to adjust your spine!" He giggled and gently placed me on the floor feet first. After he put me down I noticed that he was breathing very heavily—he had a severe lack of endurance. I also noticed that he flicked his neck back and forth to try to work out a kink that may have resulted when he lifted me off the ground. His strength was on target for his quality of life as he aged, but his endurance and structure were not. And one, without the other two, is out of balance. All three are important to quality of life as you age.

STRUCTURE WITHOUT ENDURANCE AND STRENGTH

A healthy structure is important to quality of life as you age. On a strictly mechanical level, it certainly makes sense that proper alignment and balance is necessary for healthy bones, muscles, and nerves. If you want to stand up straight, maintain flexibility, and have balance, stability, and control over your own body, then

ESS Story: Roger Craig

Roger Craig is another great professional athlete whose commitment to the ESS principles of The 100 Year Lifestyle made a huge difference in his historic NFL career. A key member of the 1980s San Francisco 49ers team that was named "Team of the Decade," Roger won three Super Bowls and made the playoffs in every one of his eleven years in the league. He pioneered the concept of the all-purpose running back in many ways by becoming the first player in NFL history to rush and receive for at least 1,000 yards in the same season. He was also the first running back to be elected to the Pro Bowl as both fullback and halfback, and he remains the only running back to lead the NFL in receptions in a single season and to receive for over 100 yards in a Super Bowl.

Roger was a pioneer in his training also, by incorporating all three elements of The 100 Year Lifestyle—Endurance, Strength, and Structure—into his fitness routines. When he arrived in the NFL in his rookie year, he received great advice from a mentor of his, Walter Payton, who said to Roger, "Never lose your endurance." Roger took Walter's advice to heart and maintains that same attitude today running nearly forty miles per week at the age of forty-nine.

Strength training was also a key element of Roger's success and durability. Roger performs strength-training exercises

One of my good friends, Mike Epstein, owns a Gold's Gym in Paramus, New Jersey. He is an avid exerciser and works very hard on his endurance and strength training. For years, however, he's been neglecting subtle problems and irritations in his spine. While his wife and children included chiropractic care and a healthy structure as a part of their lifestyle, Mike just did the endurance and strength portion of this plan. I'll never forget the day he called me in agony. Mike "threw his back out" and was in severe and excruciating pain. Fortunately, his chiropractor got him on track and got his spine healthy again so that he could get back in the gym and continue his 100 Year Lifestyle plan. You can be sure that he now incorporates all three aspects of the ESS training into his lifestyle so that he maintains the stamina, strength, and healthy structure for a lifetime.

with and without weights to keep his body physically strong, toned, and looking good.

Since he was in fifth grade, Roger has made taking care of his structure, spine and nervous system, a priority. He grew up in Davenport, Iowa, which is the home of Palmer College of Chiropractic, where Roger and his family would go for their regular chiropractic adjustments to keep their bodies aligned and balanced. He continued the structural element of his training at the University of Nebraska where he was named an Honorable Mention All-American.

When he got to the NFL, Roger became a pioneer by bringing chiropractic treatment to many of his teammates, including superstars Joe Montana and Jerry Rice. Their visits to chiropractor, Dr. Nick Athens, were initially met with resistance by the 49ers medical staff. The players knew the importance of the care they were receiving as it kept their bodies aligned and balanced and their nerves firing on all cylinders. Just like we saw in Terry Schroeder's example at the Olympics in Chapter One, chiropractic care has now become a key component of the majority of professional sports teams' and athletes' lives.

The balance of the ESS "was definitely a key reason for my durability as an athlete and I believe it is a key reason why I am still healthy and in the best shape of my life today, even after football," says Roger.

good structure—which includes your spine, your feet, and the rest of your skeleton—becomes even more important.

A healthy structure is about much more than the mechanics alone. There is a vitalistic component as well. Here's why: Your nervous system runs through your spinal column and controls and coordinates the function of every cell, tissue, and organ of your body. For you to be healthy these nerve pathways must be free from interference and have good communication between the body and the mind. This allows for maximum function and is essential for optimum health.

A healthy spine and nervous system is absolutely essential to good health and quality of life as you age, but if you ignore the other elements of the ESS, it won't prevent you from having a heart attack or from needing to be pulled out of a chair when you are older. About a year ago I was asked to speak to a group of colleagues at a seminar. As I was talking about The 100 Year Lifestyle and the importance of getting your ESS in shape, I realized how badly some of my colleagues needed to hear this message. It's not just regular folks who need to learn and incorporate the ESS into their lives, it's doctors and health professionals as well. For years many of the leaders of this group had been taking impeccable care of their structure while also letting the rest of their health deteriorate. Several of them were anywhere between thirty and fifty pounds heavier than they should have been, and I noticed during my talk that three of them had just recently gotten out of the hospital due to heart conditions.

All three—Endurance, Strength, and Structure—are important if you want to ensure quality of life as you age. Having one or two of these is just not enough. In fact, the weakest area in your ESS training will become the limiting force in your life. The good news though is through the ESS training of The 100 Year Lifestyle Workout you will easily be able to implement a fitness plan that includes all three. So get started now to ensure your ticker keeps ticking, your muscles keep lifting, and your structure keeps standing and functioning to its full potential and works for you over the course of your entire lifetime.

GET YOUR ESS IN SHAPE: SPECIFIC WORKOUTS

To develop these ESS sequences, I worked with two of my favorite personal trainers, Dave Kenyon and Todd Cioffi. Both Dave and Todd are National Academy of Sports Medicine Certified Personal Trainers who have been studying The 100 Year Lifestyle. Dave oversees the personal training at three Gold's Gyms in Fishkill, Poughkeepsie, and Newburgh, New York, while Todd is one of the head trainers at the Gold's Gym in Paramus, New Jersey. Their passion for making a difference for their clients is extraordinary and these ESS sequences are a great starting point for beginners, a great template for intermediates, and a great challenge for advanced exercisers.

The following pictures will show you the exercises that are listed in each of the workouts that follow. Become familiar with them before you try to do them, especially if you are a beginner or you haven't worked out in a while. Once you scan the photographs and read the explanations, choose the workout that applies to your goals, whether it is weight loss, lifestyle, or performance, and give it a go. If you need further assistance, you can make an appointment with a personal trainer or log into www.100yearlifestyle .com where there are descriptions and videos of these and many more exercises online.

Strength Exercises

Choose a weight for these exercises which you can do 8–10 reps to build muscle mass, or 12–14 repsto tone muscles, with extra effort required on the last few reps. Concentrate on having good posture during all of these exercises. During free weight exercises with barbells, it is good to have a workout partner or a spotter nearby in case you need assistance.

● ●

Hip and Leg Exercises

Body weight squats—Stand in front of a bench or a chair (facing forward with bench/chair behind you) with your feet shoulder width apart standing, bend at knees until buttocks touches the bench and then stand up straight again to complete the rep—don't sit on the bench. Down 2 seconds, up 2 seconds, equal time up and down.

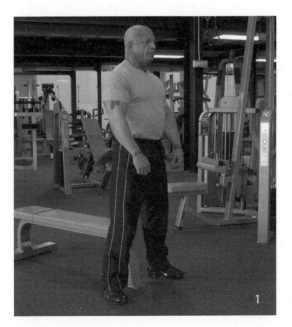
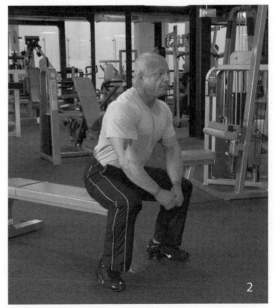

Weighted Squats (with dumbbells) *(Legs)*—Follow the instructions for body weight squats, but use weights heavy enough to cause moderate exertion on the last 2–3 reps.

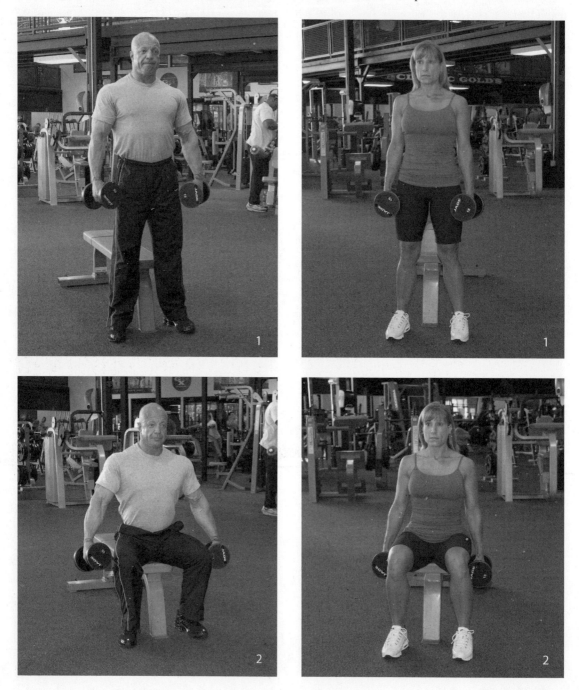

Barbell squats—This advanced squat is the same as the weighted squats on previous page, holding barbell behind neck—choose weight that is 50–60 percent of your body weight and work up from there. Make sure your lower back is straight and eyes are looking at ceiling. Keep your motion slow and controlled.

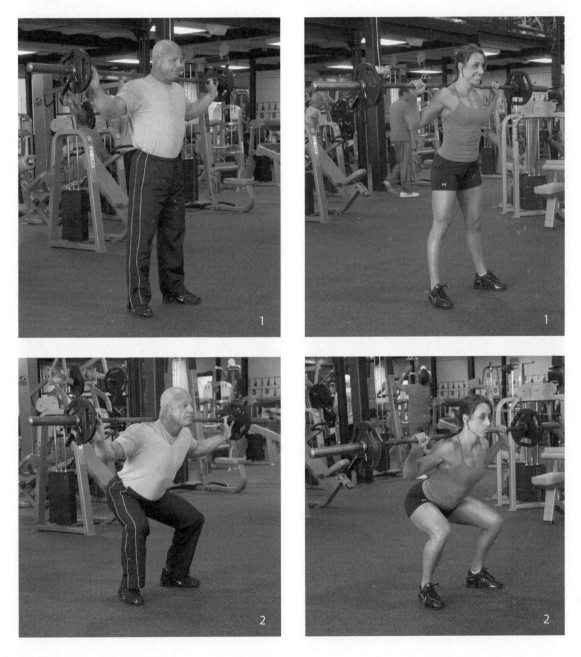

Assisted lunges—Stand up straight stabilizing yourself with a chair, bench, or railing by your side. Step backwards with your left leg while keeping your right foot flat on the ground until your left knee is just above the floor. Hold this position for 1 second and then stand back up straight again. Repeat movement with the other leg.

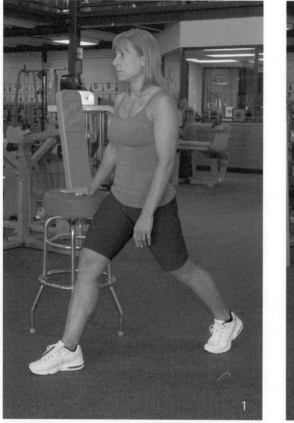 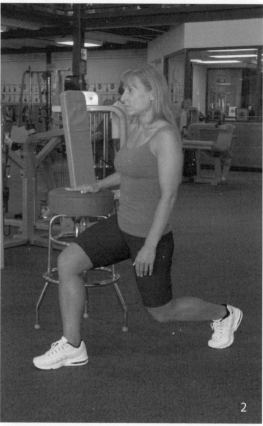

Body weight lunges (same as assisted lunge)—Without holding onto anything or stabilizing your-self, let your body's core do the work for your stability.

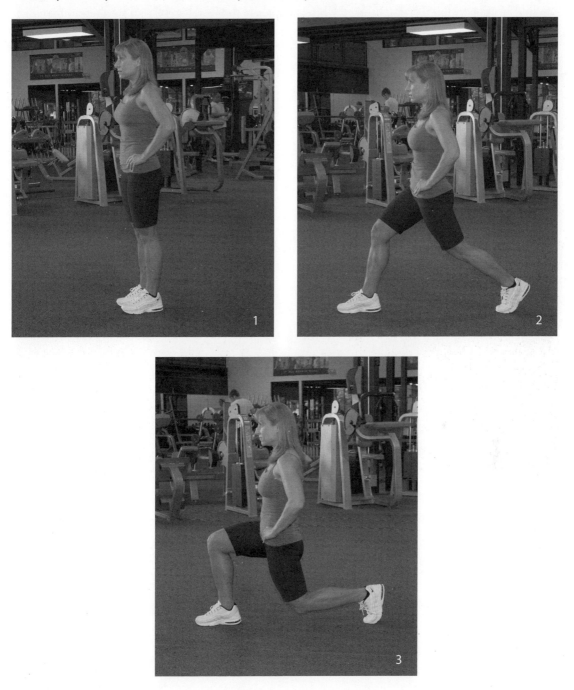

Side-to-side lunges—Lunge to one side with first leg. Land on heel then forefoot. Lower body by flexing knee and hip of lead leg, keeping knee pointed the same direction of foot. Return to original standing position by forcibly extending the hip and knee of the lead leg. Repeat by alternating lunge with opposite leg.

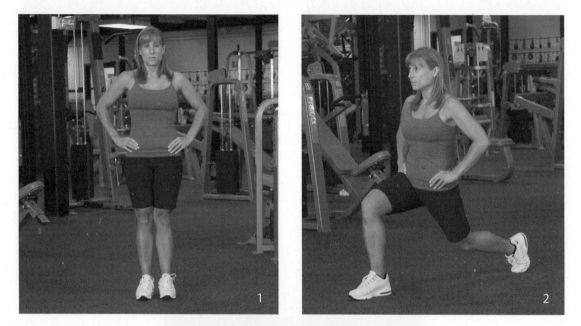

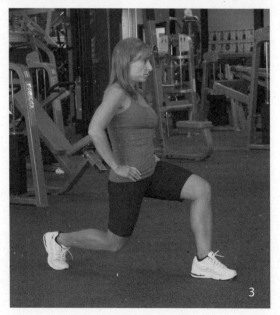

Walking lunges with weight—Hold dumbbells that are 5 percent of body weight in each hand. Start with feet together, arms at sides. Take giant steps forward until your back knee touches the floor.

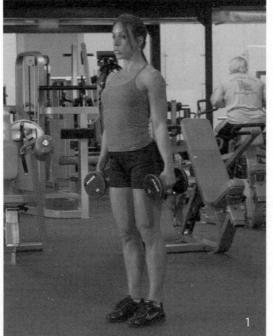

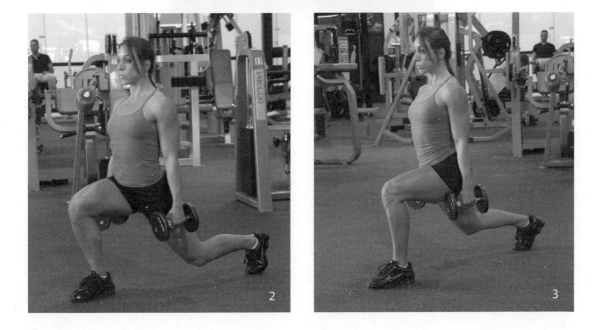

Walking–lunge twist—Stand with your feet hip-width apart. Position your arms in front of your chest with your elbows bent. With your right leg, lunge forward about three feet until your right thigh is parallel to the floor and your left knee is nearly touching the floor. At the same time, twist your upper body ninety degrees to the right. Twist and step back to start, then repeat, stepping with the left leg and twisting to the left. That's one rep. Sink low into the lunge but don't let your front knee extend past your toes. Keep your chest up and your back straight as you twist.

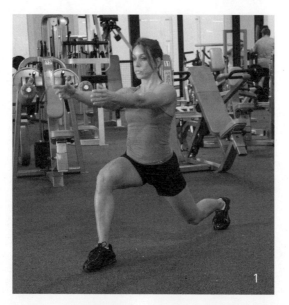

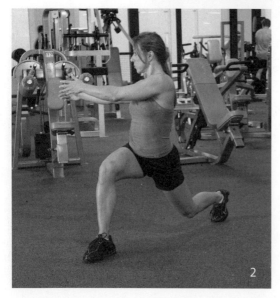

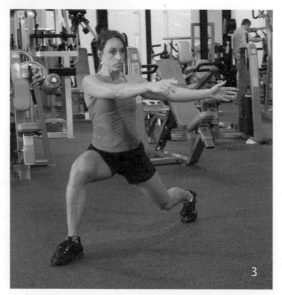

Split squat with dumbbell curl and press (alternating) *(Biceps/shoulders/legs)*—Stand with dumbbells grasped to sides. Extend one leg back. Squat down by flexing your other knee and the hip of your front leg until the knee of your rear leg is almost in contact with floor while at the same time curling the dumbbells using your biceps and then pressing dumbbells above your head and returning to original standing position by extending the hip and knee of the forward leg. Repeat. Continue with opposite leg.

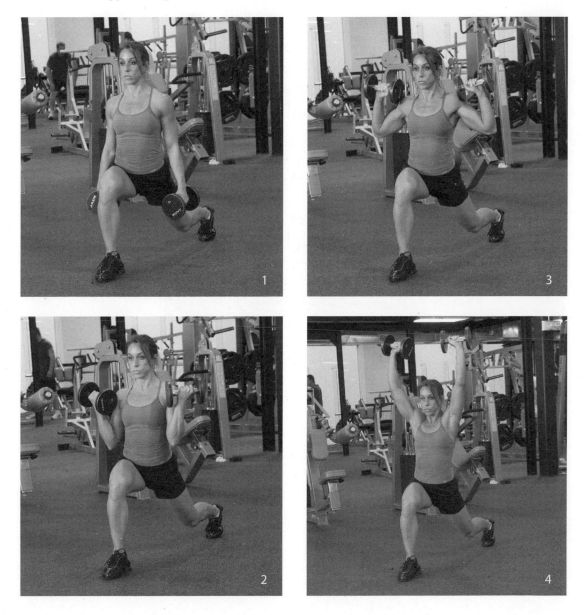

Chest and Tricep Exercises

Pushup—Lie chest-down with your hands at shoulder level, palms flat on the floor and slightly more than shoulder width apart, your feet together and parallel to each other. While bending your arms and keeping your palms in a fixed position, slowly lower your body toward the floor until your chest touches the floor. Keep your body straight and your feet together. Keep your legs straight and your toes tucked under your feet. Once your chest touches the floor, straighten your arms as you push your body up off the floor. Keep your palms fixed at the same position and keep your body straight. Try not to bend or arch your upper or lower back as you push up. Exhale as your arms straighten out.

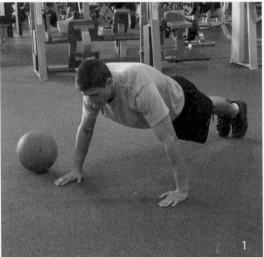

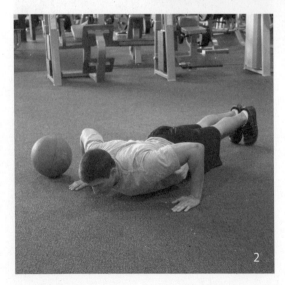
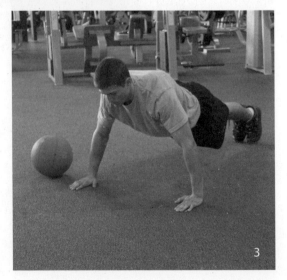

Pushups off bench or wall—This pushup, not pictured, is an easier version of the previous pushup. With your body straight, standing on your toes, place your hands a little more than shoulder width apart and leaning against a wall or a bench. Bend your arms, lowering your chest toward the bench or wall and then straighten them again to complete a rep.

Pushups using a BOSU ball—This pushup, also not pictured, is a little more challenging than the regular pushup because rather than placing your hands on the wall, the exercise is performed with the bubble side of the BOSU ball on the ground and your hands on the outer edges of the flat platform, making sure they are directly under your shoulders. Maintain a flat back, tighten your abdominals throughout the workout. Descend until your chest is very close to the platform, and then slowly push back up. Perform one set until you cannot go any more, making sure to keep proper form the entire time. The wobbliness of the ball makes this pushup more difficult.

Dumbbell bench press—Lie on your back on a flat bench with a dumbbell in each hand and your palms facing your feet. Start at arms length over your chest with arms extended together. Bring dumbbell down by bending arms in semi-arc so they finish next to your body at the level of your chest, so your elbows go back, then push weights up to starting position.

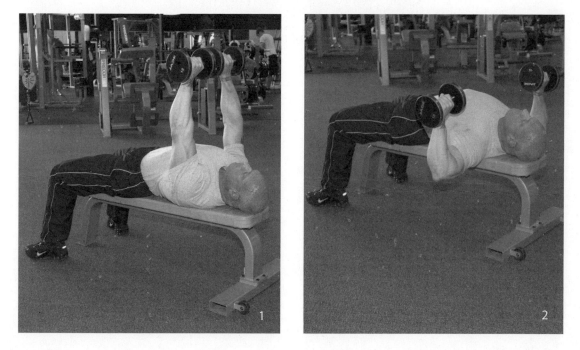

Barbell Bench Press—Lie on your back on a flat bench and your hands on a barbell. Begin with your arms extended and then lower the barbell to your chest, and then press it back up towards the ceiling.

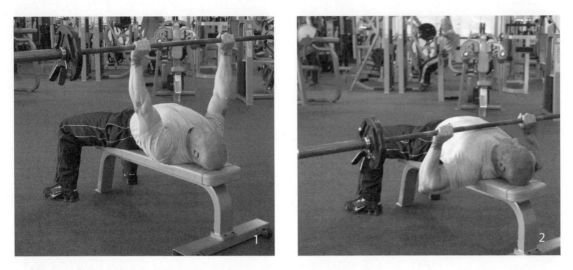

Seated machine chest press *(Chest)*—Sit on the machine, hands on the grips, and slowly push the grips out in front of your chest to full extension of arms, then slowly bring it back without bringing the elbow past the shoulder joint.

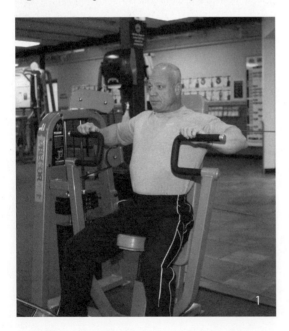 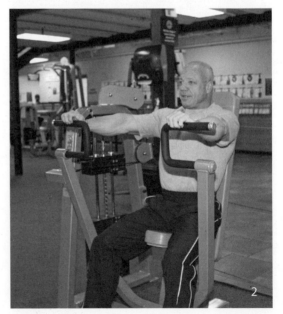

Standing cable chest press/seat cable—Stand, or sit, with your back to the weights and place a cable handle in each hand. Your hands should be at the level of your chest and your arms will be bent. Push the handles in front of you until your arms are fully extended, hold for one second and then slowly bring the handles back to the starting position to complete your repetition. Start between 10–20 percent body weight on each side to test the weight and make sure that it is comfortable for you.

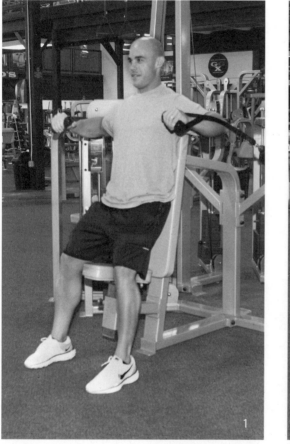 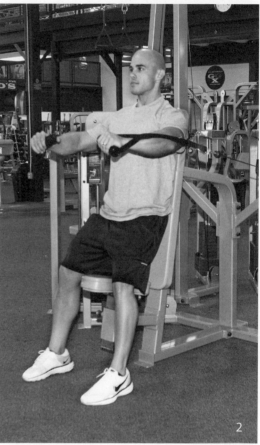

Assisted dips (*Triceps*)—Mount a wide bar with an oblique grip (bar diagonal under palm), arms straight with shoulders above hands. Press down onto assistance lever with hips and knees bent. Lower body by bending arms allowing elbows to flare out to sides. When slight stretch is felt in chest or shoulders, push body up until arms are straight and repeat.

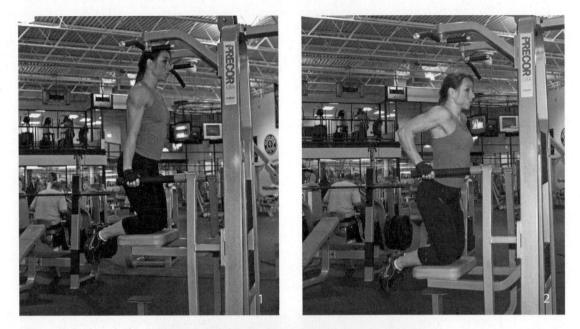

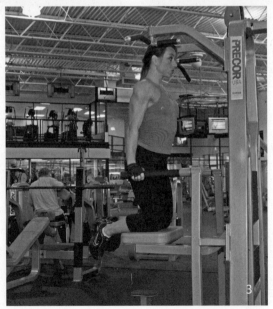

Rope push-down *(Triceps)*—For this machine stand with feet hip width apart, while holding the rope with both hands at the same time gently pushing palms to floor.

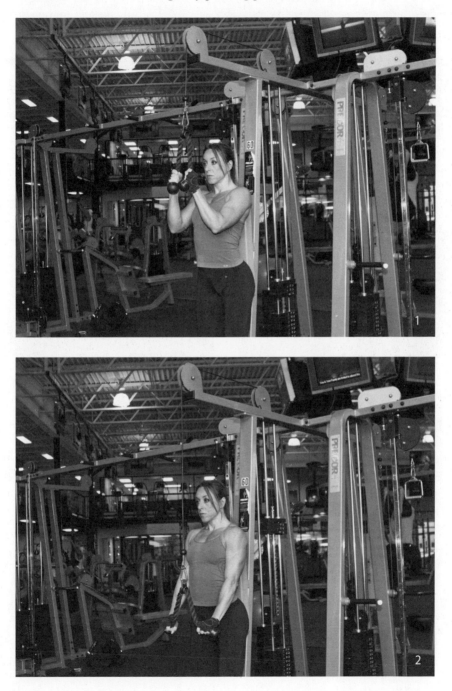

Rear deltoid shoulder exercise—rear deltoid fly machine—Sit facing the machine, grab the handles with arms extended straight, and move arms parallel to floor out to the side to finish T position.

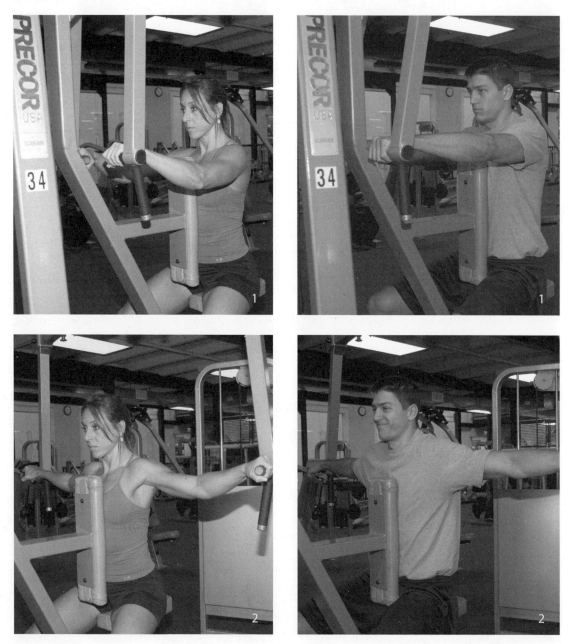

Rear deltoid shoulder exercise on stability ball—Lay face down with large stability ball on your sternum and chest. Hold 5–8 pound dumbbells in your hands held straight down toward floor until your arms are straight. Your knees should be bent slightly and toes on the floor. Keep arms straight and raise arms out and up to ceiling (forty-five degrees) to T position. Hold for 1 second at the top.

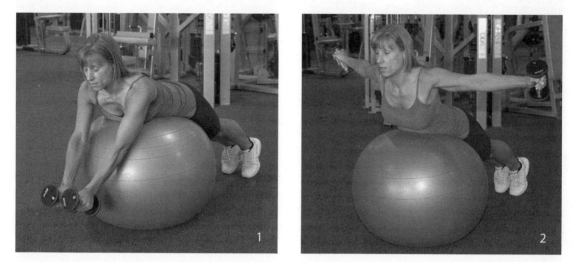

Rear deltoid shoulder exercise with dumbbell—Stand with the front of your body leaning against an incline bench or stability ball with your body at a thirty to thirty-five-degree angle. With a dumbbell in each hand, start with your arms straight down toward floor and raise the dumbbells out to each side until they are parallel to the floor finishing in a T position.

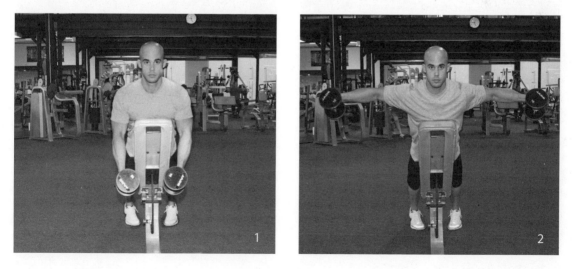

Seated dumbbell shoulder press—Sit down on a bench with your feet hip width apart, and slowly press the dumbbell above your head until your arms are straight and your elbows are almost locked out. Bring the weight back to the starting position and repeat.

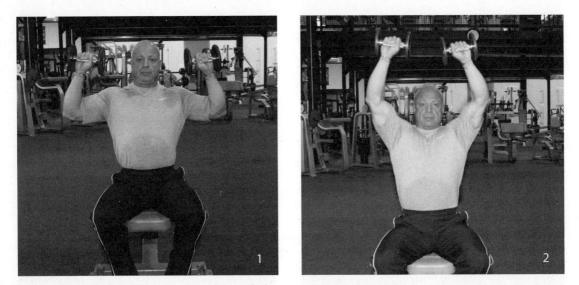

Seated medicine ball shoulder press—While seated in chair or on bench, push medicine ball above your head to straighten out arms and elbows and bring back down to rest position. If you don't have a personal trainer, start with a weight that enables you to complete the repetitions and sets below. Increase the weight to increase the intensity of the exercise.

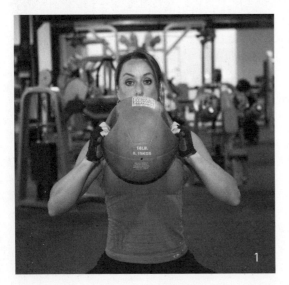

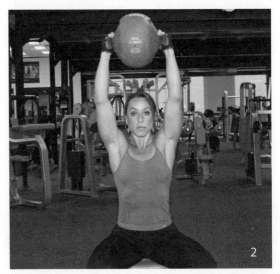

Back Exercises

Pullup (weight assisted) (*Back*)—Using machine (at first use a trainer, if possible). Stand on the platform facing the machine and grab hold of the pullup bars on either side. With your palms away from your body, slowly step onto the weight assisted bar, which will slowly lower your body until your elbows are straight and arms are extended; slowly pull yourself up, bringing your elbows slightly past your shoulders. Slowly lower back down and repeat.

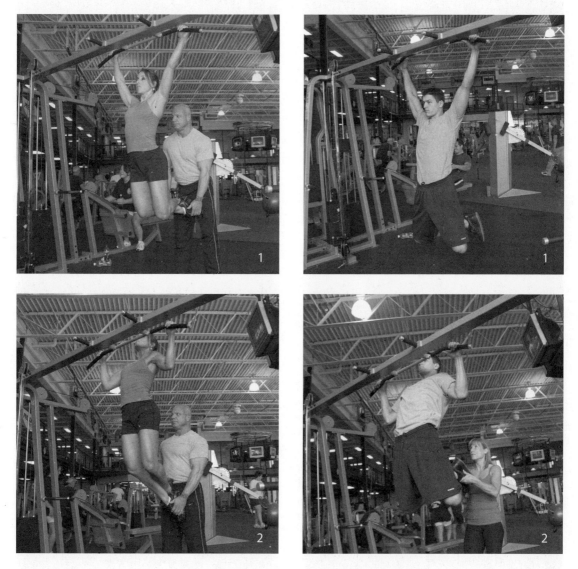

Pullups—The same exercise as the pullup above, without the assistance.

Seated row (on a row machine)—Sit with good posture (legs fully extended, slight bend in knees, arms fully extended—keep body at ninety degrees). Pull handle to belly button with elbows in and then release back to arms straight.

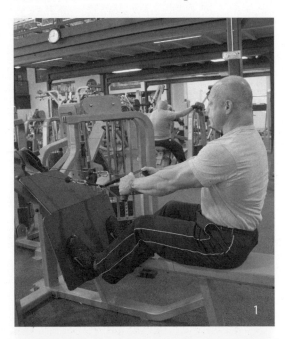

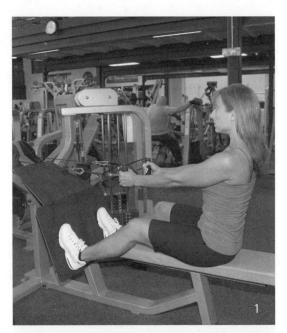

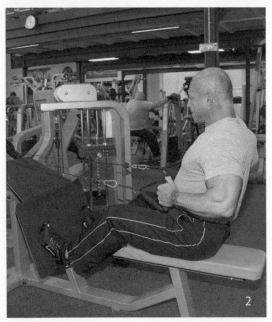

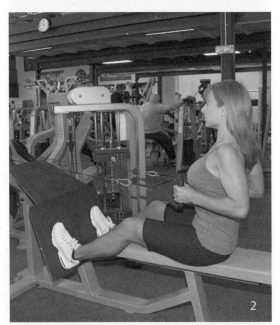

One arm bent over dumbbell row—Your left knee/hand should be resting on a bench. With your right hand holding the dumbbell and your right leg on the floor, pull the dumbbell to your right hip by lifting your elbow straight up back behind you. Hold for one second, then slowly release weight back down toward ground. Repeat.

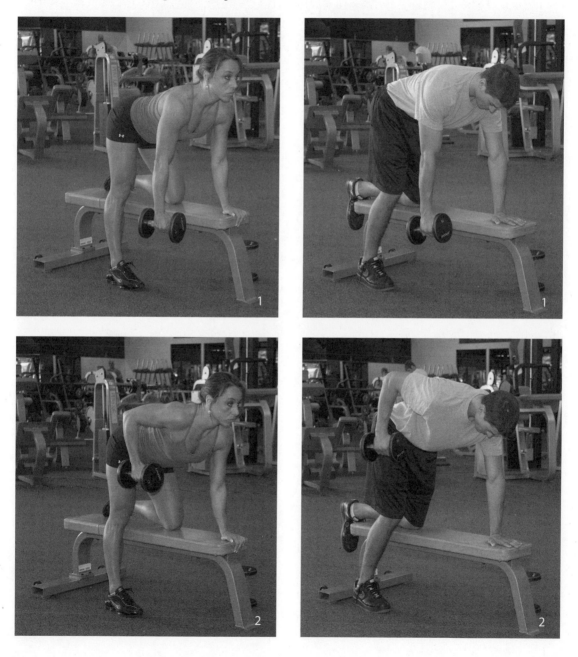

Standing cable row—Stand facing the cable machine with one foot in front of the other or feet hip width apart. Grasp two cable handles positioned at chest height, with arms straight. Pull the handles to your chest, keeping your back upright (don't lean back).

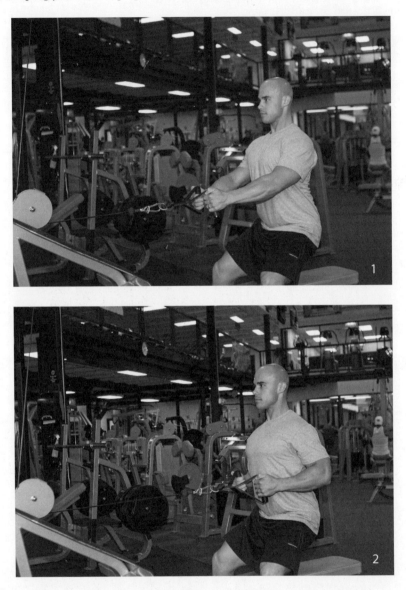

Alternating arm—see original description of cable row (one arm at a time)

Static—keep one arm back in a row position (static), while rowing with the other arm

Simultaneous—row both arms back at same time

Pushups to one-arm dumbbell rows—Lay face down on the floor and hold dumbbells in your hands in front of your chest on the floor. Start in top position with arms extended, and then lower your body so your chest is toward the floor. Extend your arms straight again; then keep one arm straight and pull dumbbell up behind you in row-type movement and then return to starting position. Push up, right row, then left row, repeat.

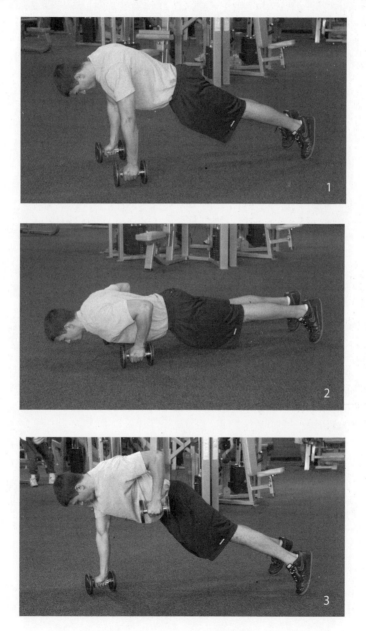

Bicep Exercises

Dumbbell bicep curl—Stand with feet hip width apart, with good posture, shoulders back, and core tight. With the dumbbell in your hand slowly flex your elbow as high as possible to the front and slowly bring weight back down until elbow is extended, keeping elbows in line with ribcage.

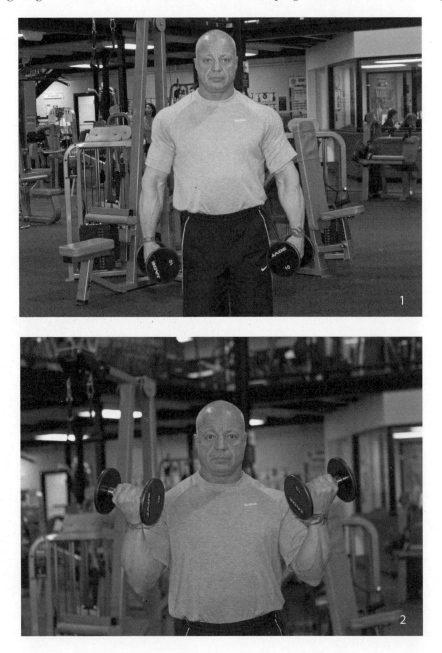

Alternating arm cable curl *(Biceps)*—Stand with legs hip width apart, holding handles in each hand (this is a machine). Start position hand at hip level; slowly bend elbow while holding on to handle. Bend upward until you can't go any higher, then gently bring it back—adjust weight according to desired resistance.

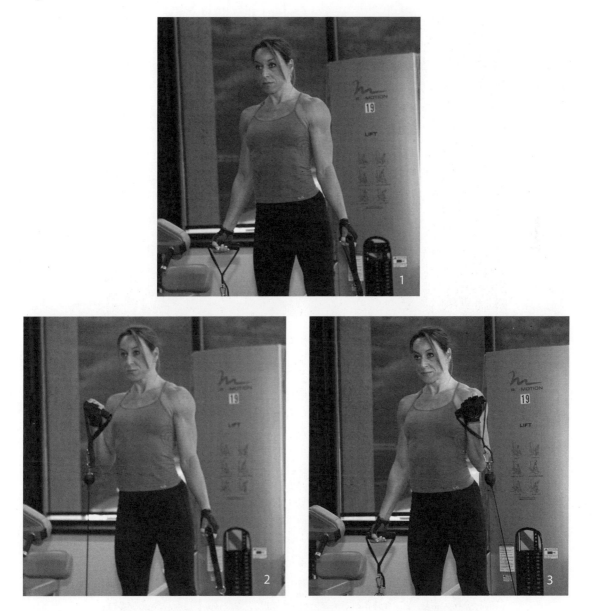

Cable bicep curl—Using a cable machine, follow the instructions for dumbbell curls.

Structure and Core Exercises

Remember: You should never feel pain during these exercises, just a slight stretch in the muscles.

Drawing in maneuver—contracting your core—laying down or standing up straight— Contract your core by sucking in your belly button and bending slightly at the waist, holding for 10 to 15 seconds then releasing.

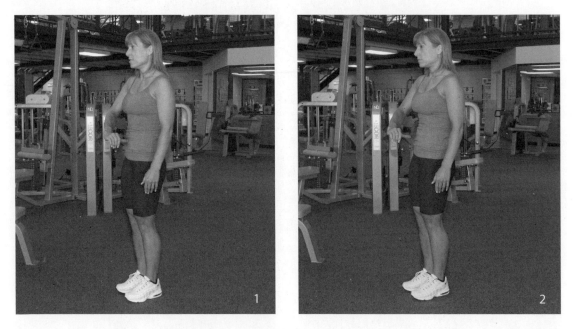

Plank on knees—face down on floor—Keep your body flat, with your knees on the ground. Prop your body up by keeping your elbows on the ground with your hands in front of them. Keeping your knees on the ground, elevate your upper body and keep your back straight. Hold for 15–30 seconds.

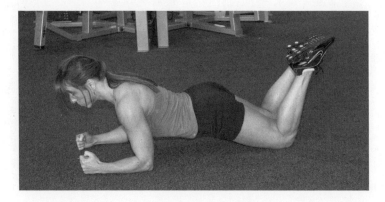

Planks (alternating legs)—Lay down in a pushup position with your body weight resting on your toes and forearms. Stiffen your body and lift your torso off the ground, with your abs pulled in tight, and pull your belly button in toward your spine. While maintaining plank, slowly alternate lifting one foot/leg off the ground at a time, keeping the leg straight. Hold for 15–30 seconds.

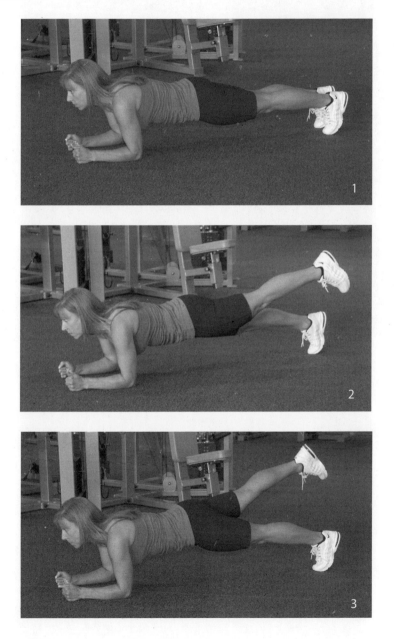

Side Planks—Lay on your right side leaning on your right elbow and forearm, and resting on your hip. Raise your hip off the ground so that your body is straight. Hold this position for 5–30 seconds.

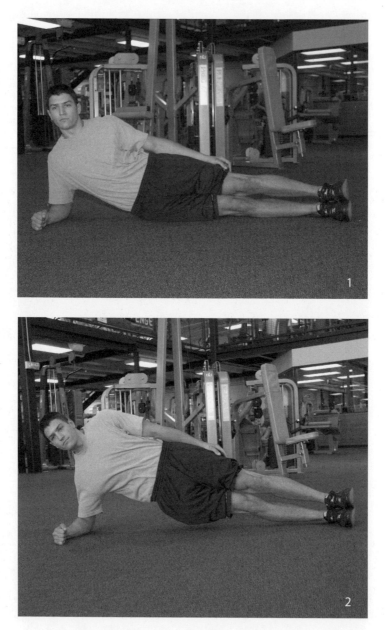

Hyperextensions—Position yourself on a hyperextension bench, beginning with the bench slightly below your hipbones and your body parallel to the floor. Flex forward at the waist until your head approaches the floor, and then hyperextend backwards toward the ceiling to complete one repetition; hold your body at the top of the movement for 1 second before beginning the next repetition.

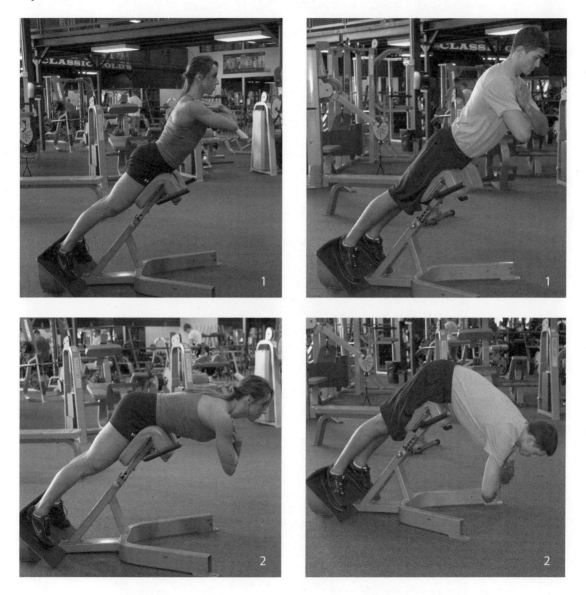

Lower back stretch—Lay face down on the floor with your hands flat under your shoulders. Push your hips into the floor and bring your chest, shoulders, and stomach off the floor. Try to look at the ceiling (not pictured). Hold for up to 30 seconds.

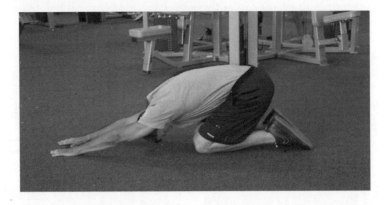

Floor bridge—Lay on your back with your hands on either side of your hips, your knees bent, and your feet flat on the floor. Raise your hips up toward the ceiling, hold 2 seconds then lower down.

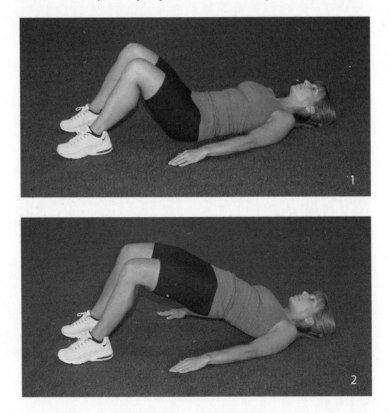

Opposite arm/opposite leg points (aka "Supermans")—Lying face down with your arms over your head, alternate raising opposite arms and opposite legs.

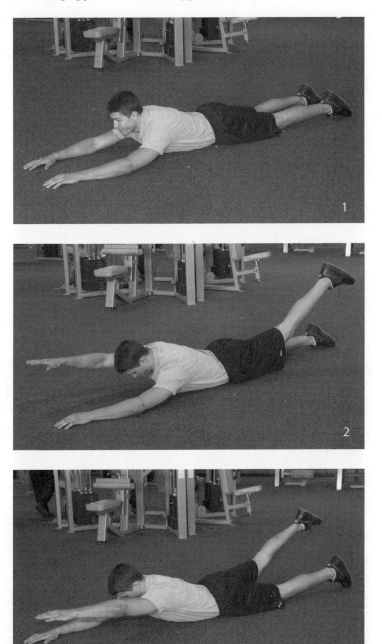

Hanging leg raises—Hang from a bar (pullup position) and raise your knees to your chest and then release back down to straight legs.

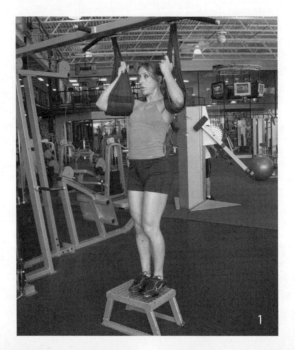

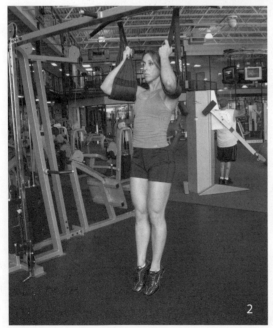

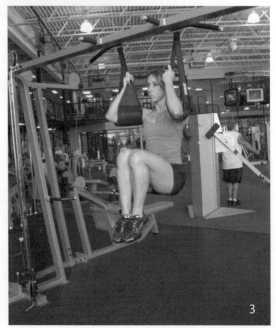

Hamstring stretch—Stand in front of a bench, keep your left foot on the ground, and place the heel of your right foot on the bench. Keep your left leg slightly bent and your right leg straight, bend over at the waist and try to touch your right hand to your right toe. Stretch as far as you can and then hold this position.

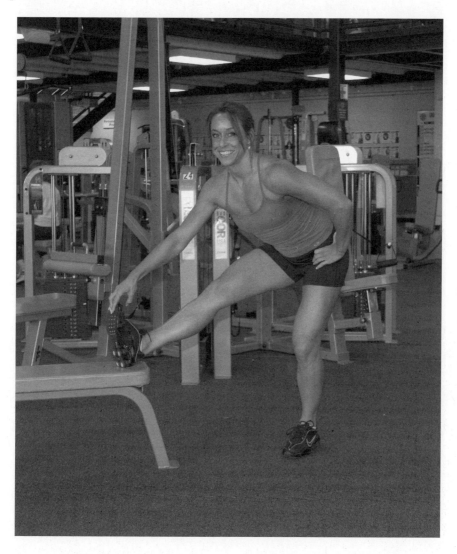

Active hamstring stretch—This variation of the hamstring stretch, not pictured, is a great dynamic stretch for your hamstring muscles. Sit on a bench with one leg on the bench extended straight, toes pointed to ceiling. Gently, slowly reach down and try to touch toe. Slowly come back to start position and repeat. Hold the stretch at the toe for 2–3 seconds then relax and release muscle.

Quadriceps stretch—Stand straight and stabilize yourself with a railing or chair in front of you. Reach behind and grab your left foot, while keeping your right leg straight and your right foot on the ground. Hold for up to 30 seconds. Switch sides.

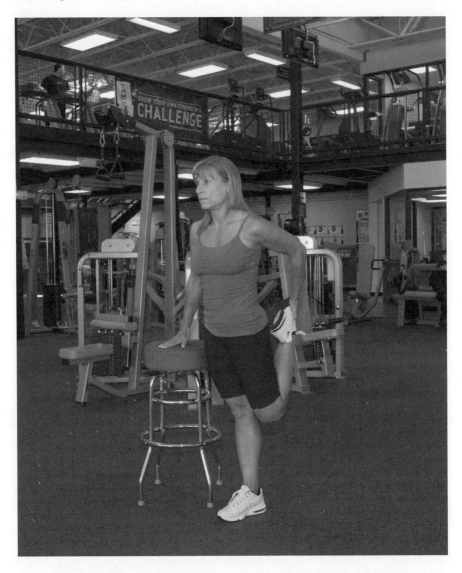

Active quadriceps stretch—This variation of the quadricep stretch, not pictured, is a great dynamic stretch for your quadricep muscles. Place the front of your lower leg and foot on a bench, facing down. Gently sit back on your foot and lean backwards, hyperextending your hip. Hold out 2–3 seconds and come back forward, relax, and repeat.

Scorpion stretch—Begin with your hands, knees, and toes on the ground, your arms straight and your back flat. Arch your back by raising your head and right leg up to the ceiling while you let your stomach drop towards the floor. Return to the neutral position and repeat with your opposite leg.

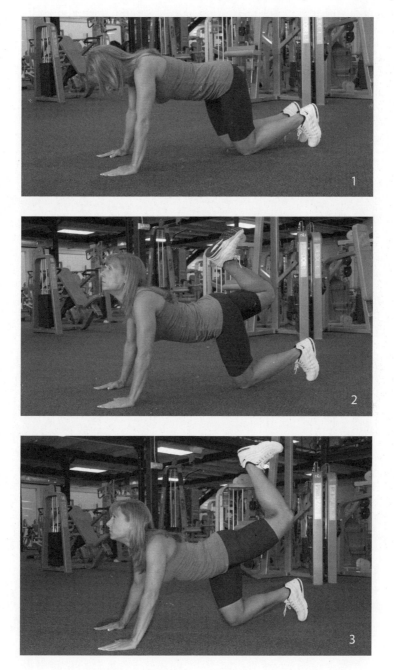

Abdominal floor crunches—Lie face up on the floor or on a soft surface, bend your knees, and bring your feet close to your buttocks. Fold your arms across your chest, or place them behind your head, and tuck your chin into your chest. Lift the upper body toward your thighs with abdominal muscles while keeping the lower back on the floor. Lower shoulders and upper body slowly and with control.

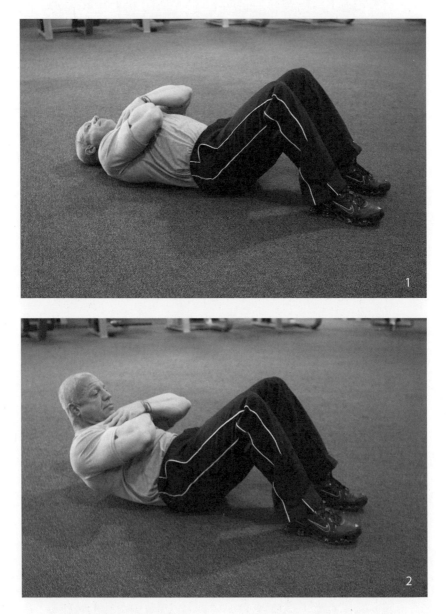

Side-to-side crunches—Lay face up on your back with your knees bent, feet flat on the floor, and your hands folded across your chest. Curl up and try to bring the opposite elbow to touch opposite thigh (right elbow to left thigh).

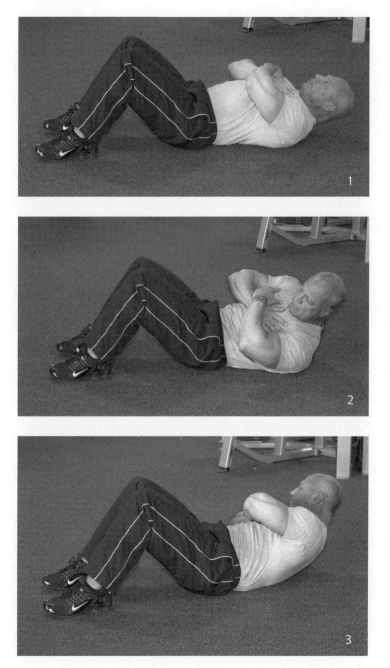

BOSU abdominal crunch—Begin by lying on your back on the BOSU ball. Keep your knees bent and shoulder width apart, and place your hands behind your head or crossed in front of your chest. Pull your abs in tight and crunch up toward the ceiling, then return to the starting position completing as many repetitions as you can.

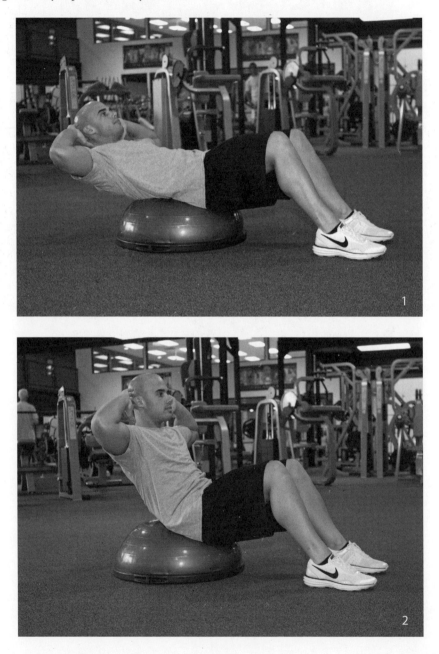

Hand walking (forward/backward)—Keep your feet flat on the floor, legs hip width apart. Lower your upper body with a stiff back without bending knees until palms are flat on floor. Slowly walk your body down into a pushup position or stiff-armed plank position. Keeping hands on floor and elbows in a locked position, slowly walk your feet up to your hands without bending the knees.

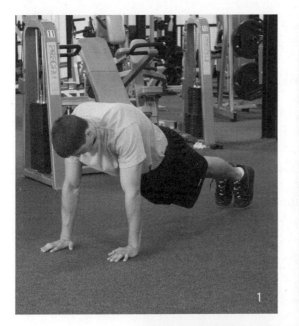

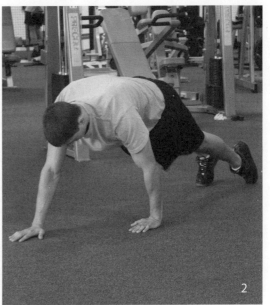

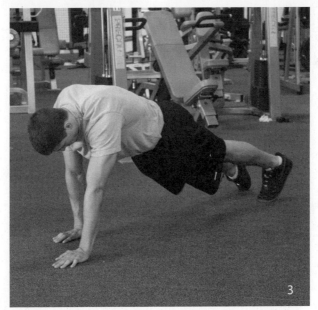

REPS are the number of times you do an exercise—for example, if you lift a weight 12 times, that's 12 reps.

SETS are the number of times you do your series of REPS—so 2 sets of 12 reps means you lift a weight 12 times, two times over for a total of 24 times.

WEIGHT LOSS: BEGINNER

This workout should take approximately 30–45 minutes.

Estimated Calorie Burn: 250 to 400 calories depending on your intensity.

Endurance

10–15 minutes of low to moderate intensity endurance training. Wear a heart monitor and exercise at 60–70 percent of your maximum heart rate. If you ever feel dizzy or light headed, stop and rest, and go see your doctor.

Do one set of each exercise with minimal rest between each exercise.

Strength and Structure

- Body weight squats (8–14 reps)

- Seated row (8–14 reps)

- Assisted lunges (8–14 reps on each side)

- Rear deltoid shoulder exercise—rear deltoid fly machine (8–14 reps)

- Drawing in maneuver (8–14 reps)

- Plank on knees (5–30 seconds, 3 reps)

- Hamstring stretch (5–30 seconds, 3 reps)

- Quadriceps stretch (5–30 seconds, 3 reps)

- Lower back stretch (5–30 seconds, 3 reps)

- Pushups off bench or wall (8–14 reps)

- Seated medicine ball shoulder press (8–14 reps)

- Floor crunch (8–14 reps)

- Floor bridge (8–14 reps)

WEIGHT LOSS: INTERMEDIATE

This workout should take approximately 40–60 minutes.

Estimated Calorie Burn: 350 to 500 calories depending on your intensity.

Endurance

From 20 to 30 minutes of moderate intensity endurance training, such as running on the treadmill or using the elliptical machine, achieving a maximum of 60–80 percent of your maximum heart rate.

Strength and Structure

Do these exercises as a circuit with no rest in between. Do a full circuit; then take a one-minute rest. Do the entire circuit two times.

- Weighted squats (8–14 reps)

- One arm bent over dumbbell row (8–14 reps on each side)

- Body weight lunges (8–14 reps each leg)

- Rear deltoid shoulder exercise (8–14 reps)

- Dumbbell bench press (8–14 reps)

- Hyperextensions (8–14 reps)

- Drawing in maneuver/contracting your core (8–14 reps)

- Full plank (hold 5–30 seconds, 3 reps)

- Side-to-side crunches (8–14 reps on each side)

- Active hamstring stretch (8–14 reps per leg)

- Active quadriceps stretch (8–14 reps per leg)

- Lower back stretch (hold 5–30 seconds, 3 reps)

- Pullup (weight assisted) (8–14 reps)

- Squats (with dumbbells) (8–14 reps)

- Standing cable chest press/seat cable (8–14 reps)

- Alternating arm cable curl (8–14 reps)

- Rope push-down *(Triceps)* (8–14 reps)

WEIGHT LOSS: ADVANCED

This workout should take approximately 40–60 minutes.

Estimated Calorie Burn: 500 to 700 calories depending on your intensity.

Endurance

Complete 30 minutes of high intensity endurance training achieving a maximum of 70–80 percent of your target heart rate.

Strength and Structure

Circuit training—Complete a full circuit with minimal rest in between circuit stations; do 2 sets for each machine.

- Barbell squats (8–14 reps)

- Pushups to one-arm dumbbell rows (8–14 reps)

- Walking lunges with weight (8–14 steps on each leg)

- Rear deltoid shoulder exercise on stability ball (8–14 reps)

- Pullups (8–14 reps)

- Hyperextensions (8–14 reps)

- Drawing in maneuver—contracting your core (8–14 reps)

- Planks, alternating legs (8–14 raises per leg)

- Hanging leg raises (8–14 reps)

- Opposite arm/opposite leg points (aka "Supermans") (8–14 each side)

- Active hamstring stretch (8–14 reps per leg)

- Active quadriceps stretch (8–14 reps per leg)

- Standing cable chest press (8–14 reps)

- Standing cable row (8–14 reps)

- Planks (hold 30 seconds)

- Pushup (8–14 reps)

- BOSU abdominal crunch (25 reps)

- Opposite arm/opposite leg points (aka "Supermans") (8–14 reps)

LIFESTYLE: BEGINNER

If your basic goal is something other than weight loss, try the Lifestyle Workouts. If you're looking for lifestyle improvement such as increased energy, personal confidence, and even high performance you will love them. The basics of the weight-loss workouts apply, but we've tweaked the overall plan here to meet your needs a bit better. The goal here is to move at the "speed of life" comfortably.

Many of the exercises here are the same as those in the weight-loss section, except that the reps, sets, and rests don't need to be done in the circuit style. Do 2 sets of each before going to the next exercise. For each exercise, do 15 reps, and rest for 30–45 seconds in between each set.

Endurance

Complete 10–15 minutes of cardiovascular exercise at low to moderate intensity. Optional endurance exercises include walking on a treadmill or riding an exercise bike three times a week.

Strength and Structure

- Body weight squats (15 reps)

- Seated row (15 reps)

- Assisted lunges (15 reps)

- Rear deltoid shoulder exercise—rear deltoid fly machine (15 reps)

- Drawing in maneuver (15 reps)

- Plank on knees (hold 5–30 seconds)

- Hamstring stretch (hold 5–30 seconds)

- Quadriceps stretch (hold 5–30 seconds)

- Lower back stretch (hold 5–30 seconds)

Optional Exercises

- Seated machine chest press (15 reps)

- Seated machine shoulder press (15 reps)

- Dumbbell bicep curl (15 reps)

- Pushups off wall *(Chest)* (15 reps)

LIFESTYLE: INTERMEDIATE

The same principles of the beginer Lifestyle Workout, only it's time to increase your intensity. This is a great workout that will exercise your body without putting excessive strain on your body. You will work up a nice sweat without getting too sore or uncomfortable. Three sets of each (same style) not circuit style, 30–45 seconds rest in between each set.

Endurance

Complete 20–25 minutes of cardio at moderate intensity. Once again, your options are many and include the stationary bike, treadmill, elliptical, running, hiking, or a sport like basketball or racquetball. Cross training (varying the type of exercise) is a great idea and will keep your workouts fun and interesting. Exercise at 60–80 percent of your target heart rate.

Strength and Structure

- Weighted squats (8–14 reps)

- One arm bent over dumbbell row (8–14 reps on each side)

- Body weight lunges (8–14 reps each leg)

- Rear deltoid shoulder exercise (8–14 reps)

- Dumbbell bench press (8–14 reps)

- Hyperextensions (8–14 reps)

- Drawing in maneuver/contracting your core (8–14 reps)

- Full plank (hold 15–30 seconds)

- Side-to-side crunches (15–20 reps on each side)

- Active hamstring stretch (8–14 reps per leg)

- Active quadriceps stretch (8–14 reps per leg)

- Lower back stretch (hold 15–30 seconds)

Optional Exercises

- Standing cable chest press (8–14 reps)

- Standing cable row (8–14 reps)

- Seated dumbbell shoulder press (8–14 reps)

- Cable bicep curl (8–14 reps)

- Cable tricep extension (8–14 reps)

- Plank (hold 15–30 seconds)

- Floor bridge (8–14 reps)

- Abdominal floor crunches (15–20 reps)

LIFESTYLE: ADVANCED

The goal with this workout is to move through life with a greater level of energy and intensity.

This workout is more intense, will require an hour to complete, and will be more demanding on your body. You will definitely need to work up to this program and your level of concentration during your training will have to increase. When you get to this level, your ESS will be in shape and you will enjoy getting the most out of your body.

Complete the full circuit three times with 1 to 2 minutes rest between circuits.

Endurance

Complete 30 minutes of high-intensity cardio training; track your heart rate throughout. You can power walk with weights, run, bike, or hike outside, or you can use the AMT, elliptical, treadmill, stationary bike, rowing machine, or play basketball, racquetball, or any other sport that increases your heart rate. Make sure you wear your heart monitor. You can vary your endurance training to keep your heart rate up for the entire workout, or you can mix up your training with intervals by elevating your heart rate for 2 minutes and then lowering your heart rate for 2 minutes. Your maximum heart rate should be 70–80 percent of your target heart rate.

Strength and Structure

- Barbell squats (15 reps)

- Pushups to one-arm dumbbell rows (15 reps)

- Walking lunges with weight (each leg) (15 reps)

- Rear deltoid shoulder exercise on stability ball (15 reps)

- Pullups (15 reps)

- Hyperextensions (15 reps)

- Drawing in maneuver (15 reps)

- Planks alternating legs (15 reps)

- Hanging leg raises (15 reps)

- Opposite arm/opposite leg points (aka "Supermans") (15 reps)

Optional Exercises

- Standing cable press (15 reps each)

  1. Alternating arm

  2. Static

  3. Simultaneous

- Standing cable row (15 reps each)

  1. Alternating arm

  2. Static

  3. Simultaneous

- Planks (hold 30 seconds)

- Pushups off floor and/or BOSU ball (15 reps)

- BOSU abdominal crunch (15–20 reps)

• •

High Performance ESS Training

If you are an athlete who is committed to high performance ESS training, no matter what your age, you will love the exercise options on www.100yearlifestyle.com. You can create a very sport-specific workout plan to help you reach your goals. Go there now and customize a program specifically for you.

Working Out Your Abdominal Muscles

Go to the Core Crazy section of this book and add the Core Crazy routines to these challenging workouts. While the sweat beads up on your forehead, you'll have a smile on your face as you challenge yourself.

BREAKING THROUGH FITNESS PLATEAUS

Fitness plateaus can be frustrating because you stop seeing the results. When you first start a fitness program, including The 100 Lifestyle Workout, you will be excited about your higher energy level, as well as the changes you see in your body and feel in your mind. You will notice that you need less sleep and that you are more focused during the day. You will like the way your body is beginning to change shape. Maybe you will notice that you are little bit leaner in the places you want to be lean while also becoming stronger and more toned in your muscles. Seeing these results will give you feedback to keep your motivation high and your desire to continue this lifestyle change that you are making. You will find that you are talking about The 100 Year Lifestyle more with your family and friends because of these exciting changes. By becoming aware of fitness plateaus and how they affect your body and your psyche, you can continue on your journey and successfully alter your workouts and your expectations to ensure that you stay on the path that The 100 Year Lifestyle has created for you.

The first thing that you must know about fitness plateaus is that the consciousness that you bring to your workouts is critical to your continued success. Remember that if your goal is only to lose weight and not to change your lifestyle, then you will have a tendency to slip backwards when you stop seeing measurable results. You will think that you have arrived or that this is the best that you can do, the most you could lose, or the maximum result that might be available to you. This is absolutely not true.

Reconnecting with the consciousness of living The 100 Year Lifestyle means that you will continue to eat healthy because it is good for you. It means that you will continue to exercise because it is good for you. You will continue to think good thoughts, feed your mind with positive energy, shop in healthy stores, and keep your spine aligned and balanced all because it is good for you. Quality of life motivation and the desire for the gains that this lifestyle is bringing to you will need to become your primary motivation if you want to stay off the roller coaster ride that crisis motivation alone will cause.

Life-changing principle #2, change comes one choice at a time, becomes extremely important during plateaus. If you have more weight to lose or more muscle to gain, don't let plateaus blindly sneak old destructive habits and lifestyle choices back into your life. Remember change comes one choice at a time, and think progress not perfection. As you face food, workout, shopping and other lifestyle choices, remember that with each choice you can make progress toward living your ideal 100 Year Lifestyle. Remain conscious every time you are faced with a choice so that you choose your new lifestyle, even though you may have hit a wall as far as results are concerned.

If you are like most people, you will reach some type of plateau within the first thirty to ninety days of your lifestyle change. Keep the big idea in mind when you go to sleep at night and wake up each morning, so that your choices continue to move you in the direction that will support your health and well-being. Don't slip back into old destructive patterns.

Why Your Body Plateaus—Change Things Up

We have talked several times in this book about your body's amazing ability to adapt. Just as we've talked about your body's ability to adapt to starvation diets and huge weight gains, your body also has the ability to adapt to your fitness routines and your workouts.

I was recently in the gym doing a thirty-minute endurance training session, and I was exercising next to a woman who was in fairly good condition but was still around twenty pounds heavier than she wanted to be. She was frustrated because she had already lost fifteen to twenty pounds but had reached a plateau and was unable to achieve the next breakthrough she was looking for. I asked her to describe her workouts, and I was not shocked to learn that she was doing the same workout today as when she started. She was doing a twenty-minute elliptical workout along with the same machine-based circuit training that she was doing when she started her exercise routine. I talked to her about her body's ability to adapt to her workouts and that if she wanted to get the next level of results she was going to have to change things up. I suggested that she increase the Frequency, Intensity, and Duration of her workouts while also including interval endurance trainings. I also suggested that she hire a personal trainer to design a custom-made strength-training program that would tighten, strengthen, and shrink her body the way that she wanted it to look.

The key here is to change things up. I saw her again a few months later and she had broken through. Changing her routine was a key to the breakthrough.

I ran into another friend of mine at the gym who had lost nearly forty pounds by getting on the treadmill and starting slow with a ten-minute mellow exercise session and working up to a one-hour mellow elliptical session. He did not vary his heart rate, he did not do any strength training, and he did not vary the intensity of his endurance training, and so he reached a plateau with fifteen to twenty extra pounds remaining on his frame. I talked to him about changing and varying the intensity of his workouts and adding strength training to continue to improve his results. He became defensive and chose to continue to do what he was doing, even though he was frustrated with his plateau. At some point you are going to have to make the choice to either continue to do the same workouts without seeing changes or results and be frustrated about it or change your routine and start the results moving again.

This is the reason why I have given you several different options for beginners, intermediates, and advanced exercisers, and multiple options for going core crazy. This will make it easy for you to add variety to your workouts and change things up.

The 100 Year Lifestyle dotFit Me Program also includes a wide variety of exercise options for you to keep your routine fresh and fun, and prevent plateaus from knocking the wind out of your sails. Keep your routine fresh and ever changing and you will keep your motivation high for a lifetime.

CHAPTER SIX:

Go Core Crazy: Strengthen Your Center of Gravity

Let's go core crazy!

If you want to remain fit, healthy, strong, and active over the course of your entire lifetime you need to have a healthy core. Your core consists of your abdominal muscles, hip flexors, lower back muscles, and hip extensors and is the center of gravity for your entire body.

You'll hear people who have not aged well say all the time "I feel like I have gotten shorter as I have aged." There are several reasons for this. First, if they haven't taken care of their spine and kept its appropriate alignment, then the forces of gravity combined with imbalances in joint function and nerve deterioration, as well as a loss of fluid in the spinal discs, will cause a person to get shorter with age. Second, people often develop very poor posture habits, slouching while they stand or sit. This does not have to happen to you and is not a part of normal aging. Having a weak core can contribute to your getting shorter with age.

FINDING YOUR CORE

Your core is located 2–3 inches below your navel. You can find it by standing straight with your feet flat on the floor shoulder width apart, your spine straight, your shoulders straight, and your eyes looking forward. Pretend that there's a string on the top of your head that is pulling you upright while at the same time your heels are being pulled into the floor. This will give you the feeling of being stretched out, and you will probably be at your tallest height when you are in this position. Stretch your body to its limits, take a deep breath in through your nose, and let it all the way out through your mouth while contracting your abdominal muscles. Take another deep breath and do the same thing, and see if you can feel your core or your center of gravity. If fitness is new to you, your core may be hidden underneath a layer or two of fat. Don't worry if you can't find your core right now. As you participate in this program, you'll find it once again. If you focus on it and strengthen it, you'll build your strength from the inside out. We have a fun saying in the chiropractic profession that *energy flows from above down inside out.* You are beginning to experience this process as you search for your core.

THERE'S MORE TO CORE

Your core area is surrounded by numerous muscles, organs, ligaments, nerves, and of course, your spine and pelvis. That's what makes this Core Crazy program unique compared to many of the other programs out there. It takes the entire region into account. All too often you will hear a fitness professional talking about the core or abdominal area and only focusing on the muscles. That's simply not enough. The muscles are only one component of the core. And by going core crazy you will be able to strengthen and care for all of the other elements critical to keeping your core strong. Your muscles will give you the strength, but remember that muscles are attached to bones, so they depend on bone alignment for their health and their positioning for proper function. Your muscles are also controlled by nerves. When a muscle does not have the proper nerve supply it will begin to weaken and atrophy.

Here is a list of the muscles that make up your core along with the general spinal nerve supply:

Muscles: Rectus Abdominus, External Obliques, Internal Obliques, Transverse Abdominus, Latissimus Dorsi, Multifidus, Hip Abductors, Hip Adductors

Spinal Nerve Supply: The core muscles are supplied by the spinal nerves that run from the middle of the spine, approximately T6 to the base of your spine including the lumbar and sacral nerves. For these muscles to be healthy and function properly, these nerve pathways must be healthy.

CORE AND THE SPINE

People underestimate the importance of good alignment and a healthy spine and nervous system as it relates to the core and even more importantly, healthy aging. But most professional sports teams do not. I have many good friends who are chiropractors working with professional sports teams and Olympic athletes around the world, and their focus on a healthy spine and core helps athletes function at their highest level.

Unfortunately, most people only take care of their spine when it hurts, and they ignore their alignment until they have pain. This is not a good idea. Lifestyle care, which can be as frequently as one or two times per week to once a month, is ongoing care that is not symptom-based. Instead it is based on a combination of criteria such as the underlying condition of your spine, your activity level and lifestyle

goals, is a much better way to go. Especially since research in *Spine* reported that "nerve root compression can exist without pain."

The Journal of Manipulative and Physiological Therapeutics reported in a study by B. L. Rydevik that five to ten millimeters of pressure can interfere with the nutrition of the nerve, starving it of necessary nutrients. Researcher Seth Sharpless at the University of Colorado found that spinal nerve roots, where the nerves exit the spine, only took eight to ten millimeters of pressure, about the weight of a dime, to reduce nerve transmission. Another study by T. Videman, M.D., from the Institute of Occupational Health in Helsinki, Finland, found that "after two weeks of immobilization, the first signs of eburnation (scar tissue) appear in the bone." Keeping your spine healthy, aligned,

Situps Alone Won't Do It

I remember years ago I had a patient who was a fitness maniac for decades and was focused on her muscle strength and her looks without being concerned about the other elements of her core, namely the nerves and the alignment of her spine. For years, she seemed to maintain a six-pack effortlessly, until one day in the middle of a workout her lower back gave out on her. I took a standing spinal x-ray, and she was shocked to find out that at the age of forty-three she already had a deteriorating disc at L4 and L5, where the nerve supply was not only affecting her back but also her legs—the lower muscles of her core and her organs that were being supplied by that region. When she injured herself she couldn't understand how she could possibly have hurt her lower back, especially considering she'd done so much to strengthen her abdominals. Many people have a similar experience. That's because the balance of the ESS—Endurance, Strength, and Structure—is crucial to quality of life as we age. For my patient, aligning her spine and removing this nerve pressure enabled her to get back into her fitness plan while strengthening the balance of the ESS and her core.

and balanced is crucial for long-term core, spinal, and nerve system well-being. Your chiropractor will be able to determine whether or not you have pressure in your spine, whether you have pain or not.

OBESITY, YOUR CORE, AND YOUR BACK

A lot of evidence exists that confirms back issues need to be addressed. In fact, the United States alone spends nearly $90 billion a year on the treatment of back-related conditions. One of the major contributors to back issues might surprise you: obesity. It's the cause of many of the back-related pain and struggle people experience in this country, in particular when it is combined with the focus on crisis care only. That's why the self-care and health care elements of the Health Care Hierarchy of The 100 Year Lifestyle are so important. This Core Crazy

program will address some of these issues by keeping your core fit and eliminating the weight problems associated with back pain.

CORE STRENGTH FOR SPORT PERFORMANCE

All of your movements in nearly every sport are initiated from your core, so it makes sense that a strong core will make you more athletic, more stable, and stronger on every level. I recently hired a strength and conditioning coach, Tom Bender, to help my youngest son, Cory, develop his strength and soccer skills. His team was getting ready to play in the Disney Showcase tournament against the top competition in the country and he wanted to be ready. At the age of fifteen he was going through a major growth spurt. His body had grown very long and lean. He was going to need to spend some extra time

ESS Story: Tammy Koser-Loosli

My top weight was 230 pounds. I had congenital spinal stenosis and back surgery about five years ago to relieve nerve compression, excruciating back and sciatic nerve pain, and partial disability in my right ankle from nerve damage. I have worked a desk job for the past twenty years of my life and over the last couple of years I had been turning into a major workaholic at around sixty hours a week. Approximately seven years ago, with a very low calorie diet, I went from 230 pounds to 165. Unfortunately, because I was following a low-calorie diet without focusing on overall fitness and proper nutrition, I always lacked energy and experienced muscle loss along with the fat loss. I was also constantly regaining and losing at least twenty pounds—and I eventually gave up at 165 pounds. I had tried to start exercise programs off and on over the past few years, but never made it past the first three weeks due to aggravation of my spinal condition. My ESS was completely out of shape. I have wished for the body transformation that I have achieved, but until meeting with the fitness training staff at Gold's Gym, I thought that it was just that—only a wish. Now I feel great, both mentally and physically.

I met with two of the professional training staff for a free consultation—which was a real eye opener for me. They convinced me that, with proper nutrition and a realistic exercise plan, I could reach my goals—and I could do it without the severe back pain that I had been associating with exercise.

The first couple of weeks were tough. They had to convince me that I really could *and should* eat 1,600 calories day—a majority of those being carbohydrates. I couldn't register why I was being told to eat more carbs—because that's exactly what a lot of fad diets are preaching against. They also

with the ball to find his touch with his longer limbs and bigger feet, so I felt that Tom would be able to help him rediscover his new body. When Tom designed Cory's program it was 90 percent core training and agility without the ball, followed by 10 percent of the time with the ball, using the new knowledge and conditioning that he had just received. Cory's progress

had to change my mind about certain fitness routines that I was sure would throw me into another bout of excruciating back pain, brain-numbing painkillers, and downtime. I told them that jogging and me do not mix and they were crazy if they thought I would eventually be able to jog at all, let alone for thirty minutes straight. Three months later, I was jogging up to twenty minutes and eating my words. I took care of my structure. Did I mention, no back pain or sciatic nerve pain?

Through my trainer's patience, encouragement, and positive feedback, I not only have an improved body and fitness level, but an improved mindset. I am becoming more addicted to fitness and nutrition, and I am excited that I have found a lifestyle that I can live with and isn't just the latest diet craze.

I have dropped a major percentage of fat, gained muscle, improved my cardiovascular efficiency, and discovered energy I didn't know that I had. My stress levels have decreased greatly due to my improved mindset and that natural calm that I get after pumping some weights or pounding the treadmill. I have learned to make time for myself and to care for myself. My meals are balanced and I am eating the proper amount of calories at the right times to avoid sugar lows and hunger attacks. I have reduced my work-life to forty to forty-five hours per week as I have started to focus on my health, and yet my quality of work has increased as a result of a more positive attitude and increased energy levels. My back and core feel stronger for the first time in years and I can't wait to hit the water this year and actually participate in waterskiing, Jetskiing, and volleyball! I feel ten years younger and stronger, and I am ready to start experiencing and enjoying life again! I am excited about living my ideal 100 Year Lifestyle.

was amazing and his team, Alpharetta Ambush, went on to win the tournament with Cory scoring the winning goal in the biggest game of the tournament against the number three team in the nation, the Dallas Texans. Sure, you guessed it: I am a proud papa, and it just goes to show you that your core is in the center of it all, and with this program we want you to go core crazy.

I recently attended the International Chiropractors Association's annual Sports and Fitness Symposium held in conjunction with the Arnold Classic in Columbus, Ohio. It was a fantastic experience with energetic, dynamic speakers who are at the cutting edge of health and fitness in the world. This event enabled me to meet and speak with some of these sharp and innovative fitness minds.

I had a discussion about the core with the founder of Powercentering, Dr. Pete Gratale. With his Doctor of Chiropractic background combined with his fitness certifications and engaging personality, Dr. Pete has a very thorough and fun way of bringing people to lifetime exercise, and he understands the importance of the ESS model. You may have seen Dr. Pete years ago on the ESPN show *Bodyshaping*. Dr. Pete discussed a core strength and stability test, which is a great way for you to measure how strong your core really is. The test consists of eight different exercises with specific positions that are held for a given length of time. You can learn more about him at www.powercentering .com. As you strengthen your core, you will be able to move further along in the test, originally designed by Brian Mackenzie. I have added a few modifications here for you to go core crazy.

● ●

THE CORE STRENGTH AND STABILITY TEST WITH MODIFICATIONS

This core strength and stability test will determine your core strength and will help you to monitor your progress as you age. You will need a flat surface and floor mat and a watch with a second hand. You may want to have a partner with you while you take this test to time you and to monitor your posture, because cheating on your body position will only hurt you in the long run and give you false results.

Step one: Assume the basic plank position with your elbows on the ground, toes curled under, and back straight. Hold this position for 5–30 seconds, depending on your condition.

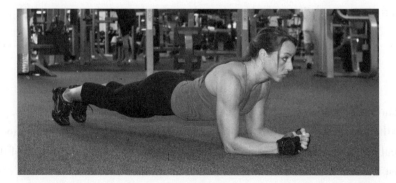

Step two: While maintaining this position lift your right arm off the ground straight out in front of you over your head, and hold for 5–30 seconds.

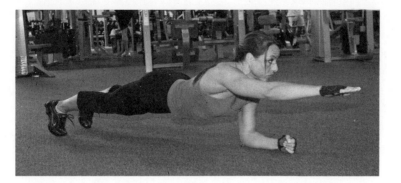

Step three: Return your right arm to the ground and lift your left arm, and repeat as you did in step two and hold for 5–30 seconds.

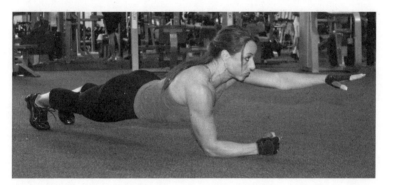

Step four: Return your left arm to the ground and lift your right leg off the ground; keep it straight and extend it straight up behind you as high as you can, and hold this position for 5–30 seconds.

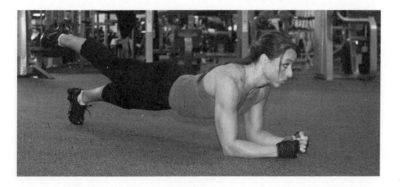

Step five: Return your right leg to the ground and repeat this motion, lifting your left leg off the ground, and hold this position for 5–30 seconds.

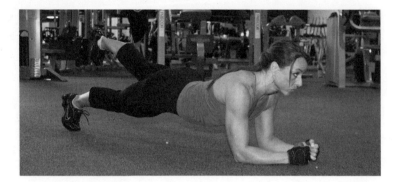

Step six: Return your left leg to the ground, and lift your right leg and left arm off the ground at the same time, holding this position for 5–30 seconds.

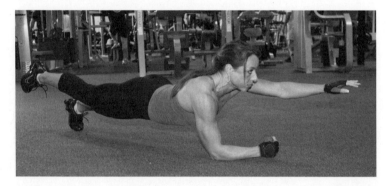

Step seven: Return your right leg and left arm to the ground and lift your left leg and right arm straight out; hold this position for 5–30 seconds.

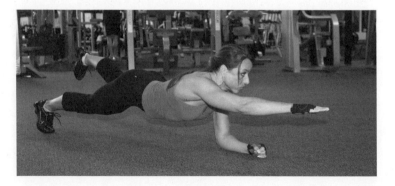

Step eight: Return to the basic plank position with both elbows on the ground, your toes curled under, and your back straight. Hold this position for 5–30 seconds.

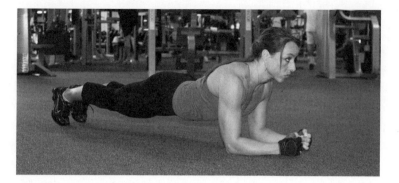

Step nine—side planks: Lay on your left side. While resting on your left elbow, raise your hips off the ground, keeping your body straight so only your left elbow and side of left foot are touching the ground. Hold for 5–30 seconds. Roll over and repeat on right side.

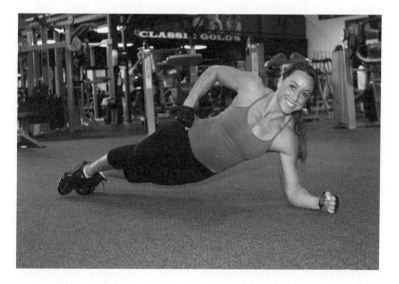

How did you do? Were you able to maintain a straight flat back throughout the entire test? Did you collapse to the ground during steps one, two, or three? Were you able to complete the entire test? Make a note indicating how far you got in this test and then retest yourself in thirty days. After thirty days continue this process and continue to test yourself every thirty days until you can get through the entire test with ease. This test measures how well you're doing in improving your overall core strength.

GOING CORE CRAZY

The Core Crazy program is made up of four routines, and as your core strength improves, you can build your way up to the different levels, which will incorporate different equipment. The beginning exercises will not use any equipment at all. As you strengthen your core, you will be able to incorporate a Xerball, stability ball, and a functional pulley-based weight system into your Core Crazy routine.

Begin by following each routine exclusively if you are a beginning exerciser. If you're advanced and perform well on the core strength and stability test, then move on to the ball programs, mixing and matching the different elements of each program to keep your Core Crazy program fun and fresh.

Wear your heart monitor when you do these routines and you'll see that you will elevate your heart rate and burn a lot of calories. Combine these Core Crazy programs with endurance training on the Precor AMT, the elliptical, the bike, or by hiking or running outside, and you will most certainly get your ESS in shape.

Core Crazy with No Equipment

Plank Variations

- Elbow plank with your legs together

- First variation—raise one leg at a time

- Second variation—raise one arm at a time

- Third variation—raise (opposing) one arm and one leg at the same time

- Fourth variation—to strengthen hips do first, second, and third variations with legs slightly further than shoulder width apart.

- Fifth variation—try it on hands instead of elbows

- Side elbow plank—start with your legs together and then raise one leg at a time, and then switch sides

Stomach Hyperextensions

First start flat on stomach with your legs on the ground and hands straight out and flat in front of you like Superman. Raise your upper body and hold for a few seconds then drop. (10–12 reps)

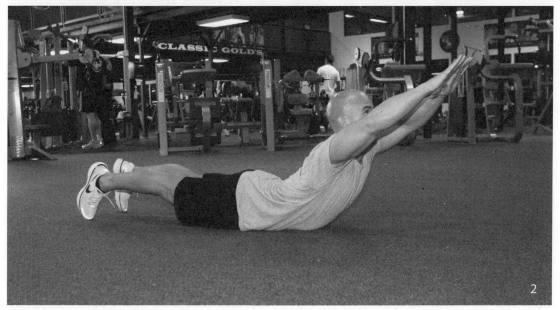

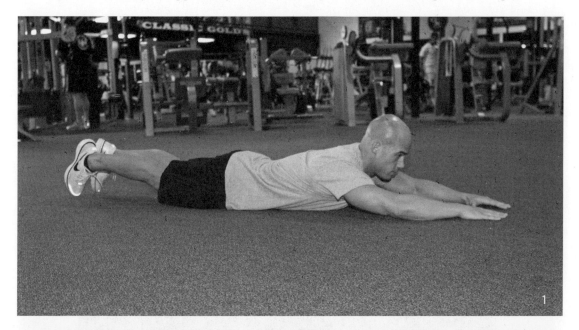

Supine Crunch

Lay on back, feet flat on the floor with your knees bent, bend hands across your chest. Roll your shoulders up contracting your core. Hold for a second then lower down.

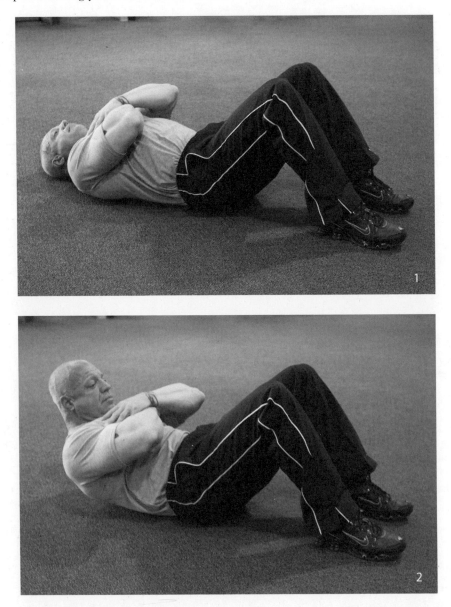

Rotational version: Rotate opposite elbow and opposite knee toward each other while raising your body up at the same time. Switch sides.

Cat's Cradle

Get on all fours (knees and hands). Arch your back down toward the floor (your stomach will point downward) and your head toward the ceiling. Then roll your hips underneath you while you arch your back up to ceiling while squeezing your core together. (10–12 reps after holding)

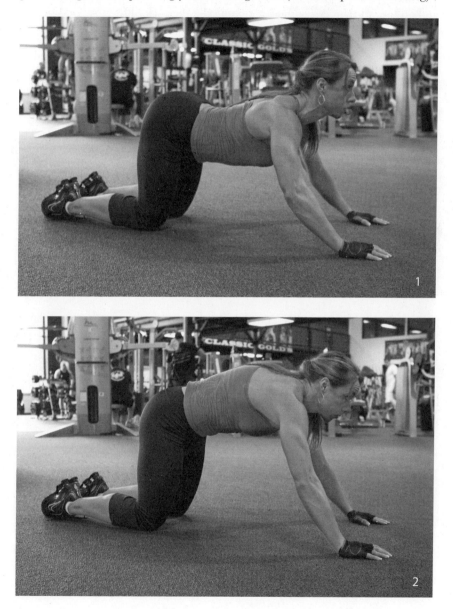

Hold: 1 second beginner, 1–2 seconds intermediate, 2–3 seconds advanced.

Core Crazy with a Weighted Xerball

Floor to Ceilings

Start standing up. Grab the handles of the ball holding it in front of your chest, bend your knees, and lower the ball toward the floor without touching the floor. Hold for 1 second then raise the ball back up to your chest, then up over your head to a full upright position, contracting your buttocks muscles when you get fully extended, and hold for 1 second. (10–12 reps)

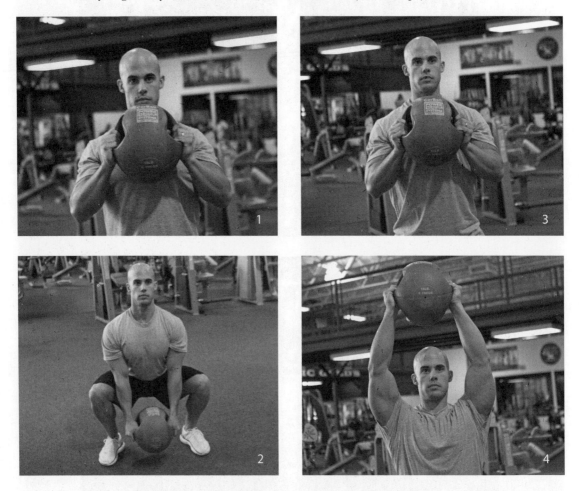

Rotational version: Begin in the same position, but take a slightly wider stance and bring the ball down to your left toe. Hold for a second and then raise up to a forty-five-degree turn in the opposite direction, bringing the ball over your right shoulder with your arms fully extended. Repeat on the opposite side. (10–12 reps)

Overhead Side Stretch

Start with the ball at your chest and your feet shoulder width apart. Raise the ball straight over your head and slightly lean to the right, while contracting your gluteal muscles to protect your back. Hold for 2 seconds then return to center. Then lean to the right and repeat on left side. Hold for 2 seconds then bring the ball down. (10–12 reps on either side)

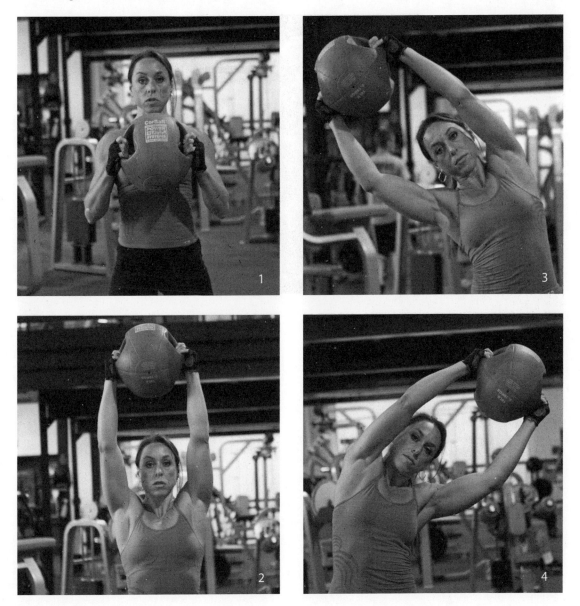

Upright Rotation

Standing up straight hold the ball at chest level, and turn to the right, contracting the opposite gluteal muscle. Hold for two seconds, turn back to the center, and then turn to the left. Keep feet flat on the floor. As a variation hold the ball three to six inches away from chest. (10–12 reps on each side)

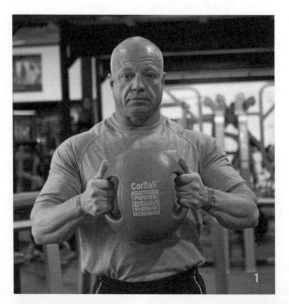

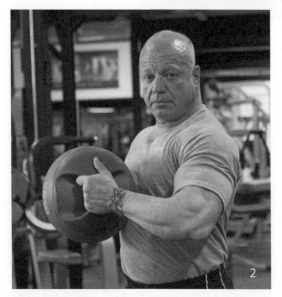

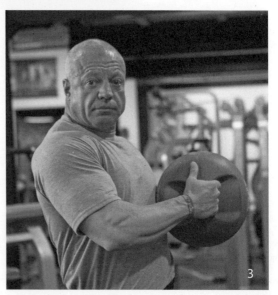

Upright Rotation Press

Start with the ball at chest level and rotate to the right while stepping with the right leg to the right, and pointing your toe in the direction you are stepping, bending your right knee and extending the arms out while holding the ball so the arms are parallel to the floor. Come back to center and repeat exercise to the opposite side. (10–12 reps)

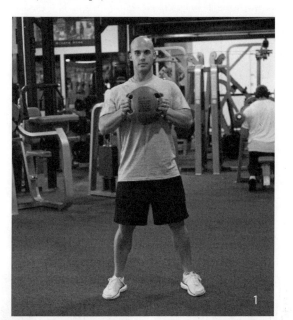

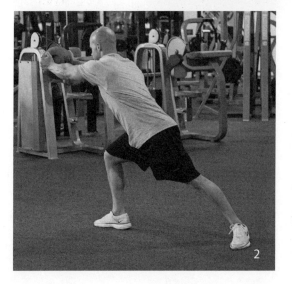

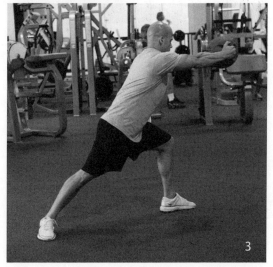

One Arm Rotation Floor to Ceiling

Holding the handle of the fitness ball, bend your knees slightly and then press the ball up toward the ceiling with your left hand. Slowly bring the ball down toward the right foot, and hold for a second. Bring the ball back up to the shoulder press area, bring the ball up to the ceiling, and turn toward that side (think *Saturday Night Fever*). Repeat on the opposite side.

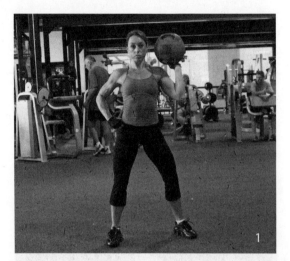

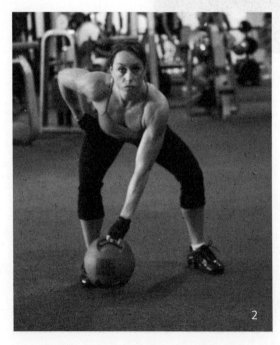

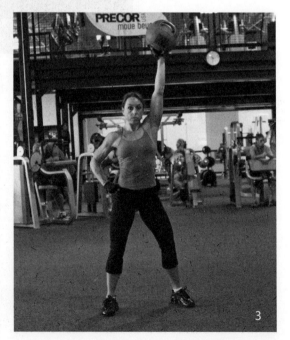

Crunches

Laying on your back place your feet flat on the floor, with your knees bent, holding the ball to your chest, and roll your body up into a crunch position contracting your core.

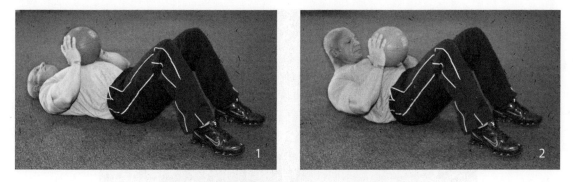

Variation one: Alternate bringing one leg up at a time with each crunch.

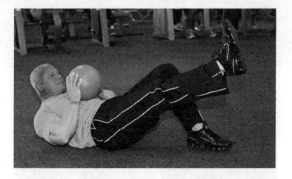

Variation two: Press the ball up toward the ceiling at the top of your crunch.

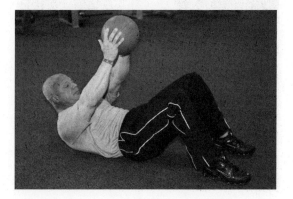

Leg Crunch Variations

Variation one: Laying on a bench hold the ball between bent knees, keep your back flat on the bench, and roll your knees up to your chest with the ball and then bring it back down. (10–12 reps)

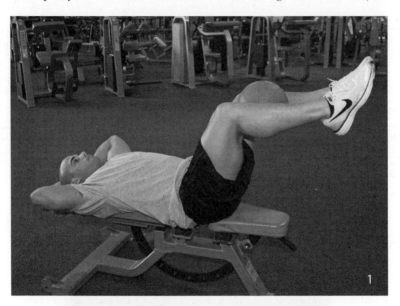

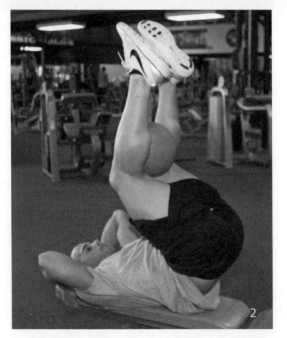

Variation two: Laying on your back, hold the ball between your heels and buttocks by squeezing your legs, raise your knees to your chest, and then bring them back down again. (10–12 reps)

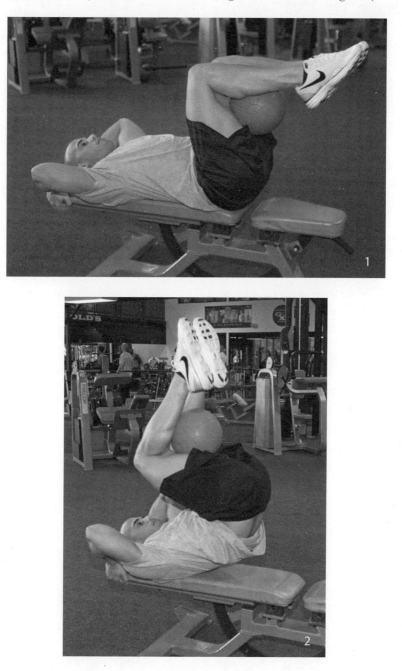

Variation three: Hold the ball between your knees rotating side to side.

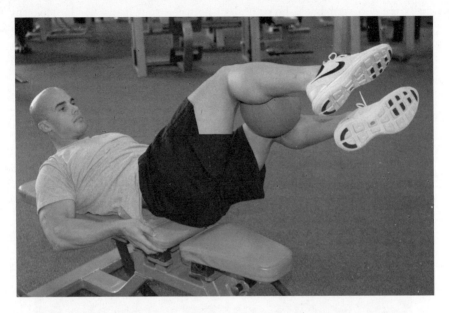

Variation four: Hold the ball between your heels and buttocks rotating side to side.

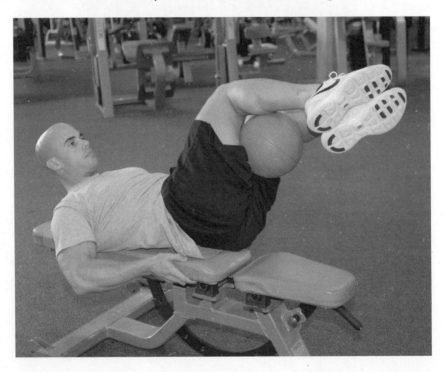

Core Crazy Stability Ball

Whole Body Roll

Lay on the ball with the ball under your core and your hands on the floor in front of the ball. Walk your hands forward until your feet are on the ball. Hold for a second and then walk your hands back until your core is on ball again. That is 1 rep. (10–12 reps)

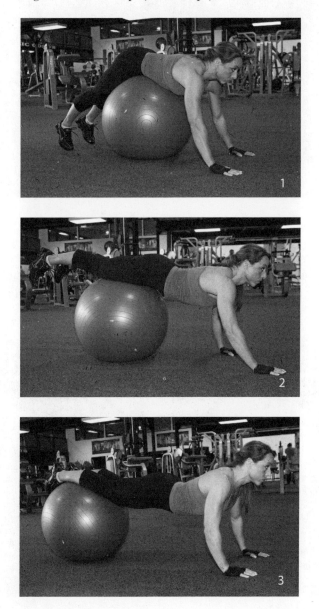

Advanced variation: When your toes are on the ball, put your body into a jackknife position (upside down v with buttocks toward ceiling) with the balls of your feet on the ball.

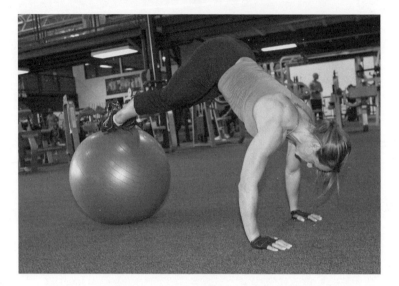

The Bridge

With the ball behind you, place your feet flat on the floor, bend your knees, and rest your upper back on the ball. Raise your pelvis up to the ceiling so that your body is parallel to the ground, hold for 2 seconds, and go back down. (10–12 reps)

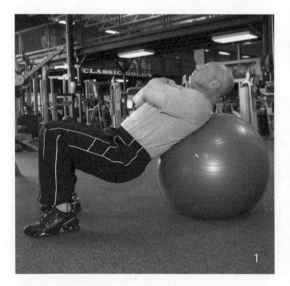

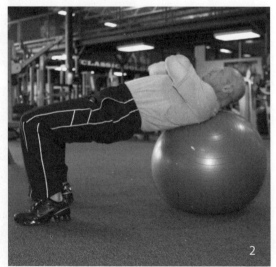

Variation two: Lay on the floor on your back with your lower legs and knees resting on the ball, and thrust your pelvis/hips toward the ceiling so that your body is straight and only your shoulders and head are on the floor. Hold for 2 seconds. (10–12 reps)

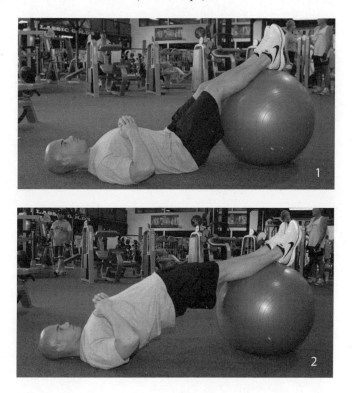

Advanced: Laying on your back with just your heels on the ball, thrust your body into plank position so that only the backs of your shoulders and head are on the floor and your heels are on the ball. Hold for 2 seconds. (10–12 reps)

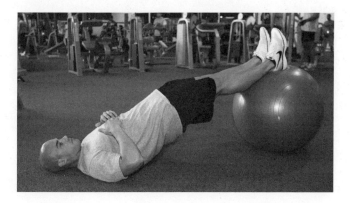

Crunches

Sit on the ball leaning slightly backwards so that your lower back is touching the ball, and recline at about forty-five degrees. While sitting on the ball form a crunch with arms across your chest and roll forward into a crunched position. Hold for 2 seconds. (10–12 reps)

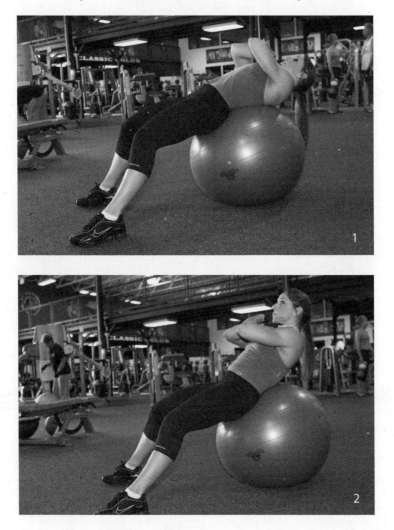

Variation one: Straighten up your hands and point them to the ceiling; crunch up thrusting hands toward ceiling.

Variation two: Alternate one hand at a time toward ceiling.

Top to Bottoms

Laying flat on a bench holding the ball above your head, simultaneously raise the ball above your stomach while you raise your feet toward the ball and grab the ball between your feet. Then bring your feet back down with the ball while you bring your hands back down over your head. Repeat this process grabbing the ball with your hands and bring the ball back over your head. This completes 1 rep. (10–12 reps)

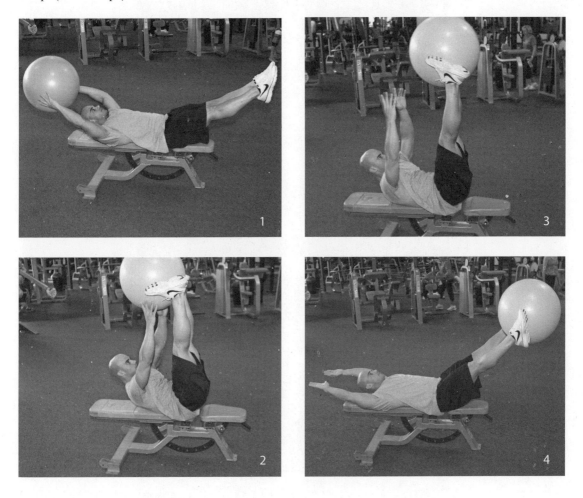

Side Bridges

Lay on the ball sideways with the left side of your core flat against the ball, your feet touching the floor, and your hands straight above your head. Roll over the ball so your hands move toward the floor, and then raise yourself up so your hands are pointed up toward the ceiling, using the side of your core to do the movement. Then switch sides so you are on the ball with your right side of your core.

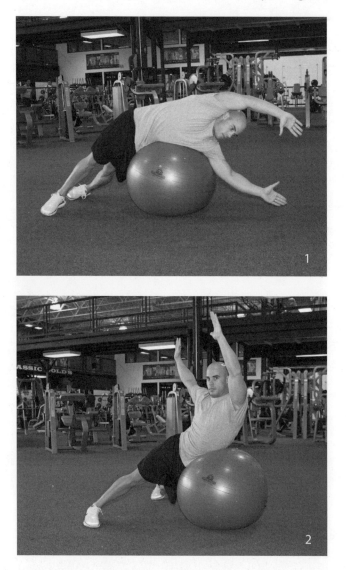

Easier variation: Fold your arms in front of your chest. (10–12 reps)

Pullup Bar Core

Hanging Knee Raises

Grab the pullup bar with your palms facing forward and body hanging; bend your knees, raising your lower legs behind you so they are parallel with the floor, and cross them at the ankles for stability. Raise your knees up to your chest and hold for 2 seconds and then lower legs. (10–12 reps)

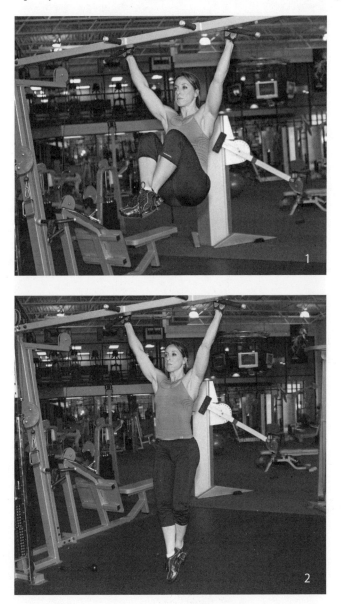

Hanging Knee Raises with Rotation

Hang from the bar in the same position as above and slightly rotate your lower body with knees to the left and feet to the right. Raise the knees up with your body slightly twisted and hold for 1 second; then drop down and repeat on the other side. (10–12 reps)

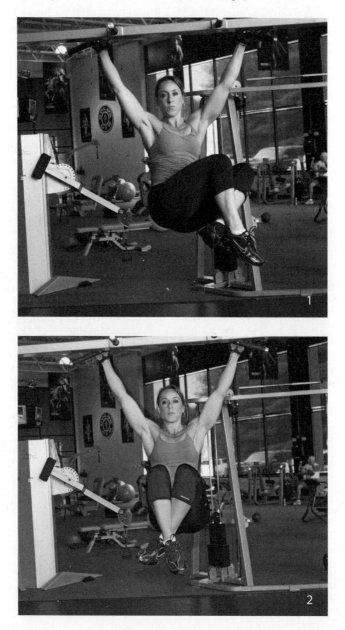

Core Crazy with Functional Training Equipment
(using pulley-based strength-training equipment)

Forehand

Stand sideways next to the machine with the pulley handle at the height of your pelvis. Stand so that your right hand is holding the pulley and your body faces forward. Slightly bend your right leg and in an explosive movement lead with your core bringing the pulley across your body with your arm extended to the outside and then release (think tennis forehand swing). Hold for 1 second and release. Repeat. (10–12 reps)

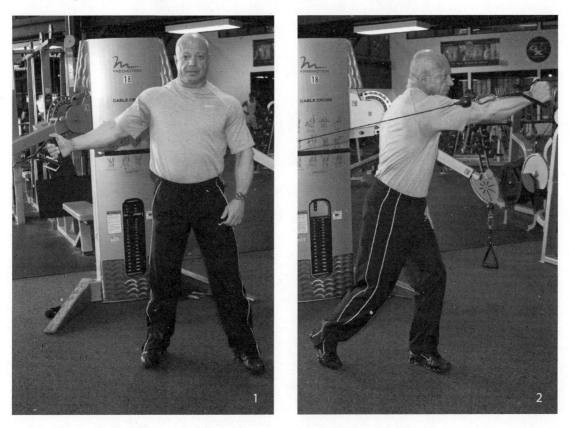

Turn around 180 degrees so your left side is toward the machine and left hand is holding the pulley handle. Bend left knee and, in an explosive movement, open hips and bring pulley across your body to opposite side, finishing with your left hand extended over your right foot. Return to starting position. (10–12 reps)

Backhand

Stand with your right side against the machine, reach with the left hand across your body, and grab pulley handle. In an explosive movement bend your right knee slightly and step out to the left, bringing the pulley across your body and finishing with your left arm extended to the side over your left foot. Then return to your starting position. (10–12 reps) Repeat on opposite side.

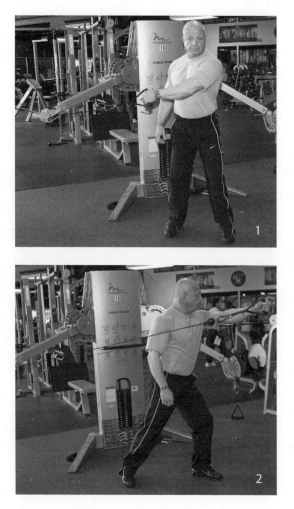

Turn 180 degrees so that your left side is toward the machine and your right arm reaches across your body grabbing the pulley handle. Leading with your core bend your left knee slightly and in an explosive backhand movement bring the pulley across your body so that your right arm is straight out toward the right side over your right foot (backhand in tennis).

Downward Chop (also known as wood chop, pile driver, or pole plant)

Stand sideways to the machine with your right side facing the machine pulley and the weight above your head. Grab the pulley with your right hand and overlap the left hand on top of the right hand leading with your core. Bend your right knee slightly in an explosive movement and chop the pulley down toward the left toe, stepping slightly with your left foot, and turn left foot out at a forty-five-degree angle. Hold at lower position 2 seconds before returning to start. (10–12 reps)

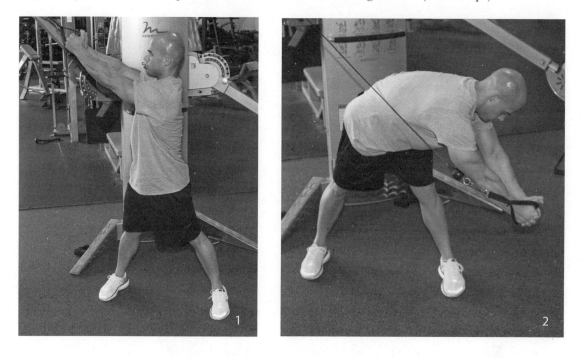

Switch so that your left side is toward the machine. Grab the pulley handle with your left hand, with your right hand slightly overlapping. Leading with your core, bend your left knee slightly, and in an explosive movement pile drive the pulley hand across your body toward your right toe, stepping slightly with your right foot and turning toe out at an approximately forty-five-degree angle and hold for 2 seconds before returning to start. (10–12 reps)

Upward Chop (golf follow-through/home run swing)

Start with the pulley down by your ankle. Stand with your left side facing the machine and bend at your knees. Grab the pulley with your left hand slightly overlapping the right. Then leading with your core in an explosive movement, bring the weight across your body and up over opposite shoulder, stepping slightly with your right foot and turning your toe at a forty-five-degree angle. Hold for 2 seconds and bring back down. Switch sides. (10–12 reps per side)

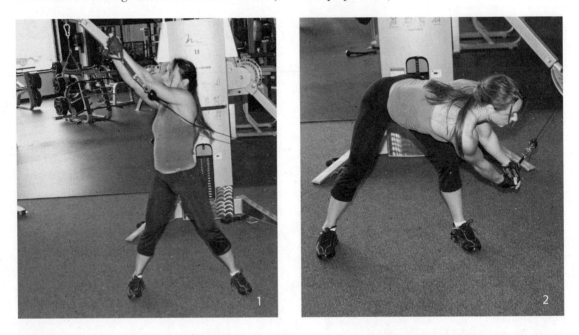

Going core crazy can be a lot of fun, but it's also a critical component of getting your ESS in shape. By combining the strength and structure components of your core, you will keep yourself lean and strong as you age.

As many people age, they tend to get soft in the middle and show their weight gain in the area surrounding their core. Implementing this Core Crazy program along with the endurance training and a lifestyle of healthy eating and good nutrition will prevent this from happening to you. You will find that your balance improves dramatically and you'll look great in a bathing suit. As you go core crazy and test your core, test your family's core as well. This is a fun way to incorporate fitness into your family's life. Get your kids, siblings, parents, and friends going core crazy. See how they do on the test and get them excited about the progress that they can make through The 100 Year Lifestyle Workout. You will have some great laughs together while you stay healthy and fit together for a lifetime.

CHAPTER SEVEN:

Put Your Best Foot Forward: The Foundation for Your Body's Structure

The 100 Year Lifestyle includes many different health and wellness components, such as nutrition, fitness, stress management, and maintaining healthy relationships. But there is a secret player in the game that has a tremendous influence on how well we age. This "secret" is so subtle it often goes virtually unnoticed and uncared for until you have a crisis. But it's time to pay some attention to it because its existence, and incredible design, actually play a huge roll in protecting your body from tons of stress, providing protection from degenerative arthritis in the knees, hips, and spine. What's the secret? What is this often neglected, critical factor in getting and keeping your ESS in shape? It's your feet. If your Endurance, Strength, and Structure are not what they should be at this point in your life, well, just look down. You might be overlooking the foundation of your being—your own two feet.

The feet are uniquely designed to hold all of your weight while protecting your knees, hips, and spine from stressful forces that contribute to wear and tear on the joints. But if you have unhealthy feet, you might end up with arthritis, pain, and stiffness. In many cases the neglect might mean you have to have surgical procedures to repair or replace the damaged joints or spinal discs.

YOUR FEET ARE YOUR FOUNDATION

If you have ever walked on the beach, you have seen thousands of footprints and no two sets are identical. Each person has a footprint that is as unique as a set of fingerprints. We all have arches of different height and shape. The strength, flexibility, cushion, and stability for the ankles, knees, hips, pelvis, and spine all come from the three arches in each foot, and they maintain the overall healthy condition of our feet. They are literally the foundation of our entire skeleton. If you look closely, you will even see minor differences between the left and right foot, which is often where the trouble begins.

> Each foot has 26 bones, 58 joints, and 107 ligaments. There are 19 muscles in each foot, and 13 muscles from the lower leg that attach to the bones of the feet, all working together in concert to provide balance, stability, and mobility. Some of the ligaments work to create the three arches in each foot.

Think of it this way: When the foundation of a house settles a little more on one side than the other, small cracks appear in various places in your ceiling. Now most people's first instinct leads them to get some Spackle and paint and repair the crack. It might look nice, but as soon as the foundation settles a little more, it will require yet another repair. This was a temporary solution to a long-term problem; the cause of the problem still exists, because only the symptom was fixed.

Lower back pain affects nearly everyone at some point in their life, some to larger degrees than others, and it is the number one reason people miss time from work and seek relief in chiropractic offices worldwide. Where does back pain begin? For many, it can be explained with the lyrics of an old song we learn in grade school, "the ankle bone's connected to the knee bone. . . ."

Based on the popularity of knee and hip replacement surgery, evidently there's a lot

We're All Connected

Here's a little test to see how little it takes for the foot to affect the hips.

- Stand up straight and place your fingertips four to six inches directly below your belt line on the sides of your legs.

- Feel for the bony bump on the side of your upper leg. This is actually the area of the hip that attaches to the pelvis.

- With your fingers in front and behind the hip bone, very slowly roll your feet to the outside like you are a bowlegged cowboy, and then roll your feet inward like you are knock-kneed.

- What you should feel is a subtle movement of the hip bone; forward when your knees are close together and backward when your knees are apart.

- Now with one foot, roll it inward and outward and see how small of a movement you can make with your foot and still feel the hip move.

It doesn't take much movement of the foot to make the hip move, does it? Can you imagine how if one hip is rotated slightly more than the other one, it creates uneven stress? It's similar to having one wheel on your car out of balance compared to the others. It develops an uneven wear pattern and eventually fails prematurely. It could be a slow leak or a blowout. We experience similar events in our lives; either we wear out slowly or we have a sudden catastrophic injury or blowout. Replacing a tire on a car is no big deal, but it's a different story when we are talking about a knee or hip or a degenerated disc in the spine. To really keep your ESS in shape, you need to keep your feet as well balanced as you do the tires on your car.

of stress settling in those areas. Those same stresses also affect the spine, but the prevalence of back surgery seems to be decreasing a little because we have discovered that surgery on the spine has limited success. We've learned how to manage the pain without surgery in many cases, but we must address structural function or we set ourselves up for long-term chronic degeneration even if we don't have pain.

Think back to the idea of the foundation of a house. Your feet serve as the foundation to your entire body. (It's interesting that the foundation of a house is called the footings.) All of your weight is borne on your feet. The strength and flexibility of the feet determine how effectively they function as shock absorbers for your knees, hips, and spine. If they don't function like effective shock absorbers, the stress has to move up in the body, first in the knees, then hips, and finally the spine.

WHY BE FOOT FIT?

The physical stress that damages your knees, hips, and spine can begin in the feet and is one of the reasons that your footprints are not identical. When we walk, our feet flatten out to absorb shock. They're designed to do so within a specific range of motion, but most people's feet flatten out too much and usually one slightly more than the other. That difference in the two feet causes stresses that twist the knee, rotate the hip, and make the hips uneven. This excessive foot motion creates damaging stresses to the ligaments, cartilage, and muscles. These same stresses are the reason we develop calluses,

corns, bunions, heel spurs, and plantar fasciitis. If you have any of those stress signals in your feet, there may be a significant deficiency in your structure, and those stressors can cause tight muscles, knots, and spasms in the muscles and stiff joints due to cartilage wear and tear. A foot, knee, hip, or spinal blowout due to neglect can sideline you from your workouts and, in extreme cases, force you to change your style of workouts forever. Proper foot self-care and health care can help you maximize the mileage you get out of your feet to a healthy 100 years and beyond.

DO A FOOT CHECK—AN EASY SELF-ASSESSMENT

Want proof that your left and right feet are slightly different? Look at the bottom of your shoes—is one more worn than the other? If it is, this may signal that your body is accommodating for unequal stress in the knees, hips, and spine. The problem is not with your shoes; it's with your feet. Do you have one pant leg that seems longer than the other one? Does one pant leg fray or wear out faster than the other one? Some people think they have a short leg when actually one arch has flattened more than the other. This flattening can lead to chronic problems with your feet, knees, and hips as well as your entire spine and nerve system. With proper care through adjustments by your chiropractor as well as custom-designed shoe inserts, you can keep your feet healthy and keep yourself bouncing around for a lifetime.

A SOLUTION FOR A LIFETIME OF HEALTHY FEET

In the late 1950s, Dr. Monte Greenawalt was one of the first chiropractors to observe and then do something about the relationship between the feet and the spine. He made an interesting observation while he had hospital privileges to make sure that his patients continued receiving adjustments during their hospital stays. One of the things he noticed was that his patients who were bedridden actually held their adjustments better than those who were able to be up, walking around.

He tried to figure out why this was so, and with continued investigation he found an answer. His research revealed that most people have a common distortion pattern in the feet called excessive pronation—an inward rolling of the feet. This rolling subsequently causes twisting motions in the knees and hips, causing an unleveling in the pelvis and distortions and stress in the spine.

As fate would have it, Dr. Greenawalt shared office space with a podiatrist, and the only available devices to address "fallen arches" at the time were a rigid podiatric orthotic made from a hard material. Greenawalt had his friend make some orthotics to address these excessively pronating feet, but something unexpected happened. His patients actually got worse! The rigid nature of the orthotics violated a basic principle of a healthy spine and chiropractic—they immobilized the joints and held them in a stressed position. Good motion gives life to every joint in the body. Locking a joint

into one position can cause stress resulting in pain, fatigue, and deterioration.

Since the feet have three arches that are designed to move and be flexible within a specific range of motion, Dr. Greenawalt came up with something that supported them all. He built the Foot Levelers' Customized Spinal Pelvic Stabilizer, which supported all three arches within the functional range of motion but blocked the excessive motion that was causing his patients to lose the effectiveness of their adjustments. The Spinal Pelvic Stabilizer simply slips into your shoe for instant, customized comfort and support. Fifty-seven years later, his legacy continues as chiropractors all over the world are using Spinal Pelvic Stabilizers to help their millions of patients keep their ESS in shape.

ARE MY FEET FIT?

If you are saying to yourself, "This all sounds good, but I really don't have any problems with my balance, my feet are in good shape, my arches look good, I don't have any corns, bunions, or calluses, I don't need to worry about my feet," well, you do. Foot dysfunction can show up in many different ways. For example, a young high school volleyball player was receiving chiropractic care for some minor lower back discomfort. She responded very well to care in that the pain was relieved for weeks at a time, but it always seemed to return. It was easy to blame it on rigorous activity, but she also suffered ankle sprains on a regular basis. A thorough evaluation of her feet revealed minor imbalances that were contributing to her ankle sprains and lower back

The 100 Year Lifestyle Custom-Made Spinal Pelvic Stabilizer

Foot Levelers and I teamed up to create The 100 Year Lifestyle SPS, a custom-made orthotic that fits into any shoe that has an enclosed heel. The special features are listed below and they can be found at nearly all of the providers' offices listed at www.100yearlifestyle.com. The 100 Year Lifestyle SPS was designed using the best attributes of Foot Levelers technology and the ESS philosophy of the 100 Year Lifestyle.

Endurance

Research proves The 100 Year Lifestyle SPS improves endurance by reducing oxygen consumption by 6 percent.

Strength

Research also shows that proper support for the three arches of the foot strengthens specific muscles of the body. The navicular correction strengthens the psoas muscle. The cuboid correction strengthens the abductor muscles. The metatarsal correction strengthens the quadricep muscles.

Structure

The patented Gait Cycle System we have designed in The 100 Year Lifestyle SPS supports the structure of the body at optimum levels. The Zorbacel in the heel reduces shock at heel strike. The Stanceguard supports the foot at full plantar contact. The Propacel in the forefoot helps your gait during toe push off to help reduce fatigue.

pain. Once her feet were supported with Spinal Pelvic Stabilizers, her ankle and lower back problems were resolved. She didn't even need to have her ankles taped anymore. The body is designed to be stable as long as it functions within the parameters of the structural design.

In situations like the one above we tend to overlook or explain away problems such as shin splints or ankle sprains as overuse or normal considering our activities, or we justify them as being hereditary. "Mom and Dad both had low back pain, I guess I just inherited it, there's nothing I can do about it." Another thing to consider is that the supporting tissues in the feet (plantar fascia) can stretch over time due to gravity and small injuries from running, jumping, and walking on hard surfaces. Once it stretches out, it cannot shorten to restore support to the arches, so it is important to prevent that stretching by keeping the foot properly aligned and stabilized before a problem arises or to at least support the already stretched tissue so the feet can function in a healthy range of motion.

ENDURANCE, STRENGTH, STRUCTURE, AND YOUR FOUNDATION

I once had a forty-five-year-old patient, a welder by trade, who walked with a severe limp. He visibly favored one knee when he walked and when asked about it, he explained that he sprained his ankle playing football in college. He received the traditional pain-killing injections and drugs and just couldn't recover fully enough to play again. Over the course of the next twenty-three years, his condition continued to deteriorate to the point that he was dependent on a dangerously large amount of over the counter pain medication (six to eight times the recommended dose) just to function with a tolerable amount of pain. He was constantly fatigued (Endurance), couldn't do many of the physical activities he previously had enjoyed (Strength), and was beginning to walk bent over and twisted as a result of the bad knee (Structure). He had been told by a specialist that he would require a knee replacement but would have to wait ten years to have the surgery because he was too young to have it at the time. He became depressed because he had been told that relief for the next ten years was hopeless.

There Is Always Hope

The welder has finally learned that stress on his entire skeletal structure was causing accelerated wear and tear. Pain was not the primary issue; it was secondary to abnormal structure and function, so I began by creating a balanced foundation, supporting his sagging foundation (flat feet) with Spinal Pelvic Stabilizers. Once addressed, his chiropractor focused on helping the tight, weak muscles and restoring mobility to the stiff joints in his spine, pelvis, and legs. Pain is a signal of dysfunction; if you restore function, the pain will disappear. And in the welder's case, it did. Something magical happened—he began to wear a smile and laugh and joke. He began to have more energy at work (Endurance), he began to exercise by walking and lifting weights (Strength), and his posture improved and he could walk without a limp (Structure). He got his ESS in shape after years of neglect and unnecessary pain and suffering. He found his hope again after years of depression and feelings of helplessness.

The effects of pain that result from our physical deterioration are far more than physical, which is why it is so imperative that you focus on your ESS. With a good foundation your health will be much easier to maintain.

WHERE TO GO FOR STRUCTURE FOUNDATION SUPPORT

There is a vast network of chiropractors in this country associated with The 100 Year Lifestyle that do a specialized evaluation of your foundation. The makers of Spinal Pelvic Stabilizers have developed a digital scanning system that allows you to evaluate all three supporting arches of your feet. This image is used to create a custom prescription for you, and I have personally worked with them to design these stabilizers with materials that will help you optimize your activity levels for a lifetime. These Spinal Pelvic Stabilizers have been shown in research

Story: A Tale of Two Women

One of my favorite examples of contrast in aging is about two ladies who were both eighty-three years old. One looked like an old lady, hunched over at the shoulders, shuffling along as she walked. She said she was "full of arthritis" and was constantly visiting one doctor or another for a myriad of aches and pains. Her medicine cabinet was full of prescriptions, many of them to address the side effects of some of her other medications. The other eighty-three-year-old came into my office complaining of soreness in her hip, because she thought she had kicked too high in her aerobics class! Her medicine cabinet contained vitamin and mineral supplements; she took care of her ESS for most of her life, maintained balance and function in her structure, and made sure her foundation was solid by proactively caring for her feet and wearing customized Spinal Pelvic Stabilizers for many years. She invested in her ESS. It has been said that the pain of discipline is far less than the pain of regret.

When considering the 100 Year Lifestyle, I think of these two ladies because each of their mothers lived to be 100. Sure there is the genetic component, but their outlook on the possibility of living another seventeen years was totally different. For one of them, it was an opportunity to participate in aerobics, swimming, and gardening for another seventeen years! For the other, the thought of it reduced her to tears in my office as she said, "I don't want to live that long." None of us know what tomorrow will bring but we do know that investing in our ESS will result in benefits that can carry us enthusiastically and energetically to 100 and beyond, and help us to maximize our quality of life along the way.

to reduce fatigue (Endurance), improve muscle function (Strength), and improve posture (Structure), in addition to many other benefits. The 100 Year Lifestyle Spinal Pelvic Stabilizer can fit into any type of shoe that has an enclosed heel, and it is the foundation to your optimal ESS. You cannot fight gravity without proper support, and the consequences of losing that fight can be devastating.

Get your ESS in shape starting today with a solid foundation, and we will see you at your 100th birthday party dancing up a storm.

CHAPTER EIGHT

Group Fitness to Great Fitness

When you think of group fitness classes, you probably think of *The 20-Minute Workout*, the *Jane Fonda Workout*, 1970's hairstyles, and leg warmers. That's because group fitness used to be one thing: aerobics. When I think back to the eighties, when I was in chiropractic college, aerobics classes were a common part of my fitness lifestyle. I really loved the fast-paced, high-energy classes and the heavy pounding beat of the music. I found it kept me in the room for an intense hour of exercise. While I enjoyed it at the time, I found the quality of the class always seemed to depend on the instructor. There seemed to be very little science or structure to the design of the class in general.

Group fitness has really come a long way. Today it comes in all shapes and sizes, and it's beneficial for people trying to get into a routine because it really works the creative side of our brains. No thinking, no counting, just a solid workout with fun music and a great social backdrop. Group fitness is a great element to add to your 100 Year Lifestyle Workout. Classes provide structured ways for you to get your ESS in shape or crank up your performance. Group classes can also use twice the amount of energy the average person expends on their own. It's more like a sport and the results can be greater.

HIGH TECH, BIG RESULTS

What's new in the booming group fitness arena now is that group fitness instructors are professionals—trained with the scientific knowledge to develop successful strategies for the design of a group program. More than in the past, people working out in classes are really seeing results in their bodies. The variety of classes available allows you to vary your workouts to fit your mood, your fitness level, and your age.

The world leader in group fitness is Les Mills, with well over 12,500 gyms worldwide licensing their programming. The fitness company has developed classes, but not in the old-fashioned way you think classes are developed—a lot goes into the development of their classes and the certification of their Les Mills

What Are Some Group Fitness Classes?

Les Mills Programs

Yoga

Pilates

Karate

Dance

Sculpt/Strength

Spinning/Indoor Group Cycling

Silver Sneakers

instructors. They have turned group fitness instruction into a profession. Classes are scientific, standardized programs, and the people behind them are doing all of the thinking for the instructors, so that they can instead focus on their coaching technique and really engage with their classes. People who take Les Mills classes get to stay in the right brain, not the left. That means they stay where they're coordinated, aware of their space, and where no thinking is involved. No numbers, no heart rate to count, because the classes are vigorously pre-tested for the members so they know what people are going to achieve. People aren't just enjoying themselves in group classes; they're getting hooked on them.

If you live near a gym or exercise studio that offers group fitness classes, it will be easy for you to discover how popular Mills' classes are. There is a Gold's Gym around the corner from my house as well as an L.A. Fitness about a mile away. Both places offer group fitness classes in the mornings and late afternoons, and the parking lots are jam packed during these times. You can walk into the gym thinking that the entire gym will be a mob scene because of how full the parking lot is, but the truth is that a majority of the people are there for the classes

Group Evolution

1960s
Stationary bike, difficult to use, boring, clunky, twenty minutes of cycling was tough to achieve

1980s
Bikes got TV or radio inputs and maybe an electronic screen to measure time or speed

1990s
Group Cycling or Spinning, great rooms, great environment, social, hardcore workout, motivating instructor, forty-five minute commitment

In another example of evolution, old-fashioned dumbbells have evolved into strength and sculpting classes like Bodypump, the world's biggest exercise class these days. And karate classes now consist of one-hour group kickboxing sweat-fests. In every one you're motivated to stay in a room and enjoy a one-hour, tested workout that gets your heart rate pumping. On your own, you can easily hop off a bike. Classes today are social and fun. It's no wonder attrition in the sixties was about 90 percent. People joined a gym—an almost miserable place to be—and then quit by the end of the year. These days, 25 percent of the adult population goes to a gym—either a private club or some other workout facility available to them. People are more conscious of how they look, and they work longer hours so they don't have time to play sports like golf and tennis. Group classes have plugged that hole.

ESS Story: Bobbi Teibel

A few times over the course of about nine years, I started working out but gave up due to either lack of time or motivation, pregnancy, or thyroid and foot surgery. Even though I was always tired, had no energy, never wanted to do anything with my kids, had low back pain, knee, and feet pain, was overweight, and hated the way I looked, I just couldn't get started. When I was about to turn forty years old, I made the decision that if I didn't do something now, I never would! So once January came around, I jumped right into my new quest to get my ESS in shape by attempting a cardio kickboxing class and seeing my chiropractor, Dr. David Moore in Clifton, New Jersey. I was still breathing when the hour-long class was over. That class was the beginning of a life-changing journey. Before I knew it, I was taking three different classes a week, a personal training session once a week, strength training on my own three days a week, and doing thirty minutes of cardio, either walking on the treadmill or completing a course on the elliptical six days a week. I started noticing that I was fitting into my clothes better and I had more energy and felt great.

After about nine months of this routine, I had lost twenty-five pounds and cut my body fat almost in half from 29 percent to 14.5 percent. Without even realizing it, I had lowered my cholesterol, which was always in the low 200's, to 178. Only a few months prior, I could barely close my size ten pants and now I was wearing size four for the first time in my life, at forty years old. I was in the best shape of my life and felt awesome.

and as soon as the classes are over, the parking lot empties out again.

Group fitness actually encourages you to go to the gym more often. In fact, according to research released at the International Health Racquet and Sportsclub Association (IHRSA) 2009 convention in San Francisco, group fitness is the number-one service or amenity that health club members are interested in. The survey of more than 2,200 health club members in the United States and Canada in February and March 2009 showed that 60 percent of club members rate group fitness as a club's most important offering—higher than any other service or amenity. And compared with global data from IHRSA, Les Mills class

In September at a routine doctor's appointment, the doctor could not believe the size of my biceps and how I had transformed my body since the last time he'd seen me. He also could not believe what he felt in my left breast. Since that day, I have been on an incredible journey.

Within days of being laid off from the health club where I was a manager for almost ten years, I was told I had breast cancer. How could this be? But because I got my ESS in shape and started living The 100 Year Lifestyle, my only thought was just do what has to be done. My mastectomy was scheduled for December 10th, five days before my 41st birthday, but really my 39th because I felt younger and had started counting backwards. During the next month, I underwent extensive testing and dealt with all the dimensions of stress in preparing for the day I would be cancer free. The day that would change my life forever was finally here.

After the surgery, I was back in the gym doing cardio after only three weeks. Doctor's orders, otherwise I would have been there sooner. Day by day, I added strength exercises to my workouts with the guidance of my trainer. I was only able to do this because of my shape before the surgery.

At no time during my one and a half year ordeal did I sit home on the couch and feel sorry for myself. I got up every day and went to the gym. I worked too hard to get where I was and cancer was not going to take that away from me. Six years later, I have earned my Hi-Brown Belt in Thai kickboxing and am still going strong.

participants attend their clubs twice as often as other members—3.4 times per week in this survey, versus an average of 1.7 times per week globally.

Another benefit of group fitness classes is that they are scheduled. Like any other appointment you can plug your group fitness classes into your calendar to be sure that you get in your workout. You can make arrangements to take these classes with friends and/or coworkers, and treating these appointments as a top priority in your lifestyle will ensure that you show up and complete them. If you are going before work or after work, make sure you pack your workout clothes so that you never have as an excuse, "I forgot my fitness stuff." Most clubs schedule their fitness classes at least a week or two in advance with many of them having the schedule set a month or two at a time. Many of the companies that design group fitness classes change their routines quarterly so that they stay fresh, innovative, and fun and eliminate the boredom that can come from doing the same classes over and over again.

GROUP FITNESS AND YOUR ESS

Now think back to ESS—Endurance, Strength, and Structure. You can find all three of these elements in the group fitness classes available today. Group fitness classes either offer some choices that focus mainly on one ESS element or combine certain elements of two or three. For example, you may find one class more heavily focused on the endurance and structure components of the ESS and less on the strength. These classes will have a tendency not to use barbells or dumbbells, the most obvious element of strength training. Other classes may focus more on strength and structure and will incorporate strength training through the use of fitness bands or movements that incorporate using your own body weight and body positions for strength training. Almost all fitness classes, especially those with a professional instructor teaching, will focus more on structure during their class and will communicate this regularly to the attendees.

Several years ago, my wife Lisa and I took yoga classes regularly at a yoga center around the corner from our home. During every class the instructor would talk about the importance of posture, balance, and a healthy structure so that

the attendees would not only get a great workout but also minimize any chances of injury. As you learn your own body and your unique fitness skills, you will be able to adapt these classes to your own structure and your own pace.

When you take group fitness classes, don't get caught up in the mindset of "keeping up with the Joneses." In your first class or two you may be self-conscious and find yourself looking around the room and comparing yourself to other people. If you are new to fitness you may grade yourself as one of the least fit people in the room. Don't let this stop you because you will find that within two or three weeks you will get your groove going and there will be other new exercisers showing up for the first time filling up the gaps behind you. In most gyms the people in your classes will be supportive and encouraging to you because many of them will remember when they were new to fitness classes. As your fitness skills grow and you become healthier, you will probably choose to pass the support on to the obvious new class attendees as you encourage them to get their ESS in shape.

ESS Elements in Les Mills Classes

Here is a breakdown of the Les Mills classes and how they incorporate the different elements of the ESS.

Endurance Training and Bigger Calorie Expenditure:

- RPM—indoor cycling

- BODYATTACK—high-energy cardio

- BODYSTEP—step aerobics

- BODYCOMBAT—martial arts

- BODYJAM—dance cardio

Strength and Best for Lean Body:

- BODYPUMP—weight training with barbells

- BODYFLOW—yoga, tai chi, Pilates

Best for Structure:

- BODYJAM—dance cardio

- BODYFLOW—yoga, tai chi, Pilates

- BODYVIVE—low-intensity cardio and resistance training

LIFE-CHANGING RELATIONSHIPS

One of the other important elements we've discussed in The 100 Year Lifestyle has to do with strong relationships. Surrounding ourselves with like-minded people boosts our longevity. Group fitness creates the opportunity for you to meet such people. It's social to work out at a set time, with a set group of people, and if you participate regularly, you'll likely make friends with others who follow a similar routine. Strong social circles help foster quality of life and longevity. It's healthy to have different networks of people in your life, so how about a network from your spinning class? You will add the social circle of your group fitness classes to your strong network of supportive relationships, many of which you will enjoy for a lifetime.

Group fitness classes provide an energetic environment that is fun but also motivating, and you'll get results. You'll also find you reach a new level of performance because you push each other as you go along. You'll have an appointment you need to keep because your friends will be waiting for you. You'll maximize your workouts because you'll have friends in the group checking up to make sure you're going, and it's always easier to stay committed with a buddy than if you are by yourself. Whether it is in a Les Mills class or a karate class, the group environment can give you the extra motivation to reach your goals. You might find that not only are you enjoying a group class, you've become addicted to it.

When my kids were younger, Lisa and I took up karate. We loved it and continued on to complete our first degree black belts. We loved the training as well as the confidence that came with seeing our improvement as time went on. We were definitely nervous our first few classes, but after a while we made lots of friends, appreciated the encouragement, and became hooked on the workouts. I'm confident that once you find the activity you like, you'll have a similar experience.

LIFE-CHANGING, RELATIONSHIP-BUILDING, AND HEART-WARMING GROUP FITNESS

A little over a year ago I was invited to speak at the Gold's Gym in Buffalo, New York. The owners, Joe and Amy Bueme, love the fitness industry, take a lot of pride in their clubs, and more than anything they love their members. In preparation for the event, Amy drove me around to look at her different clubs and meet her. It was great meeting all of these caring and committed fitness professionals, but my favorite experience was walking into the gym and seeing a line of senior citizens who were there to attend an upcoming Silver Sneakers group fitness class specifically for seniors. Amy introduced me to all of them as the author of *The 100 Year Lifestyle* and the dialogue took off like a rocket and the chitter-chatter was a mile a minute. Their enthusiasm about wanting to live to 100 and getting healthier

and younger every day inspired me once again about the importance of telling this story. One woman looked at me and said, "Dr. Plasker, if I knew I was going to live this long, I would have taken better care of myself and I would have started these group fitness classes a long time ago." I could see the tears well up in her eyes and the overwhelming emotion she expressed as she contemplated the reality of her extended life span. She said to me, "these group fitness classes have changed my life." Once again, my friends and loyal 100 Year Lifestyle readers, you and I are getting the advance notice that our parents and grandparents never received. Let's capitalize on this advance notice. Shake up your fitness by taking some group exercise classes and you will add more fun than ever to your 100 Year Lifestyle workouts.

Why Should You Mix It Up?

Change the routine on a regular basis to balance your workouts and keep your results from plateauing. Think cross-training.

CHAPTER NINE:

Travel Fitness: Keep Your ESS in Shape on the Road

Nothing can knock you off your 100 Year Lifestyle fitness plan like travel. Playtime travel, which includes vacation, poses its own unique challenges. It can be filled with an overindulgence of food and drink combined with the tendency to lie around and just vegetate. Business travel is a challenge because you're always rushing to catch airplanes and meet tight schedules. Your food choices are often restrictive, and you can't always find the ideal exercise facilities in many of the hotels that you stay in. To make matters worse, for business travelers—whose schedules include going from the car to the train to the airport to the airplane then into the new airport, to the taxi, and to the hotel and then back again—fresh air and sunshine are often left off of the itinerary.

I had a realization when I was on my initial book tour and I was flying from city to city to talk about *The 100 Year Lifestyle*. It was my third day into the trip when I realized I was on my way to serious sunshine, fresh air, healthy food, and fitness withdrawal. I could feel myself becoming deprived of energy. I was feeling grouchy and frustrated, even though I was sleeping well. It hit me one day when I had to walk outside to go from my hotel to the bookstore for a signing. The second the sun hit my head I felt a lightbulb go on. Wow, did it feel good!

I immediately began to do full lung breathing, making sure that I was oxygenating every nook and cranny of my lungs. I took the long route to the bookstore so that the sun could beat down on my shiny head and fill my body with vitamin D (I really feel sorry for those of you with hair that unfortunately blocks out those magnificent rays). Certainly too much sun is not good for you, but not enough sun can be detrimental to your health as well. And when you are traveling and spending the majority of your time in taxis, airports, and hotels, you, like most people, are not getting enough of it. You have to make sure you get outside and re-energize. I couldn't believe what an immediate difference it made for me that day.

RESTORING YOUR ENERGY ON THE ROAD

It's a simple fix. Getting some fresh air and sunshine while you travel will make you feel better quickly. These little trips outside will bring balance to your intense travel schedule that will de-stress and nourish your body with those key elements that are so necessary for your health and vitality. The quick walks and fresh air don't have to be reserved for just dinnertime—if you have the time to do it during breakfast, do it, because often your lunch or midday schedule can get thrown off by meetings. If you have the time to go outside at lunchtime, do it, because you never know what might happen during your dinner schedule. Fresh air and sunshine are priceless commodities when you are traveling.

On a nice sunny day open your hotel room sliding glass door and allow the fresh air to fill your room. Even if the weather is too hot or too cold, twenty minutes of fresh air and sunshine will go a long way to give you the nourishment you need. Take twenty minutes to sit out on the balcony and get some sunshine while you also breathe in the air. Whenever you stay in a hotel by the beach, or the mountains, ask for a room that is facing these natural wonders. Often the fresh air, the sunshine, and the sounds will enhance your experience and give you more balance. Sunshine and fresh air are free. These natural necessities will bring you the best return on your investment and give you the energy to capitalize on every other aspect of your trip.

ESS Story: Jeff Keifer

I work in corporate America, so many of my colleagues boast that we are "road warriors"—flying from city to city or driving our territory, giving presentations, working long hours, and unfortunately, eating poorly and getting very little exercise. It had started to become harder to run through the airport or get out of a compact rental car. I was always too busy to eat properly and would not only skip meals, but would overeat at those I sat down for. My weight progressively went up, my waistline expanded, and I was always tired. Obviously I was not living The 100 Year Lifestyle. I returned home exhausted and bloated from a weeklong business trip to California and knew I had to make a change or I would end up at worst with serious health issues, or at the very least I would be forced to buy an entire new wardrobe in the next size up. Neither seemed like a good option.

The biggest obstacle I faced was getting started. Beginning any type of lifestyle change is the hardest part. I knew I had to do something but couldn't decide on how to prioritize. Diet? Exercise? Both? I always thought to start on the first of the month, or on a Monday, but I would always find an excuse to put it off.

I needed to get my ESS in shape, so I began to walk. I would try to go for twenty minutes at a time—nothing fancy. Depending on the weather, I would walk outside or at indoor shopping malls. Eventually I

Calorie Burning Travel Trips

- Park your car at the airport in the furthest spot from the door and walk to the terminal.

- When you arrive at your destination, always park your car as far from your destination as possible.

- Eat at a restaurant within a mile of your hotel and walk there.

- If you eat your meals in the hotel, take thirty minutes afterwards to go for a walk prior to your next meeting.

started training with a personal trainer. I worked out three times per week and had a set time that I did my workout. This type of accountability helped me to stay on track.

It is difficult for many of us to show vulnerability. I am a very independent person and thought I could change my lifestyle by myself. Plus, I was embarrassed that I had let myself get out of shape and didn't feel good about sharing that with others. I thought I could do this alone. But I have to tell you, *allowing myself to trust someone to help me was critical to my breakthrough.* Trusting my trainer was the catalyst that got me to the next level of fitness. Eating was important so I started writing down what I ate and got my diet on track.

I was always reminded that at each meal I have a choice. Each week I got better at breaking bad habits like eating processed or fried foods.

I also made regular visits to my chiropractor. She has been very pleased with my progress and my back has gotten stronger since I began chiropractic care and exercising. I was able to get rid of a lot of belly fat, which was taking a toll on my spine and making me slouch. I also take vitamins, fish oil tablets, and manganese to help with my bones.

I have lost thirty pounds. Ten pounds changed the way people looked at me. Twenty pounds changed the way I looked at myself. Thirty pounds changed my life. I love my new lifestyle.

START YOUR FITNESS REGIME BEFORE YOU EVEN TAKE OFF

When it comes to exercise, start in the airport. In large airports, you can walk from the terminal to the gate rather than taking the tram. In a smaller airport or in an airport where you cannot walk from the terminal to the gate, you can walk up and down the terminal once you arrive at the gate. Remember you will be sitting on the airplane for anywhere from thirty minutes to five or more hours, depending on your flight. And while we are about to give you exercises that you can do while you are on the plane, you should also take advantage of the time you have to wait for departure by being mobile in the airport.

Once you reach the gate, if you have time, do a ten-minute stretching routine that includes the following exercises:

Gate Stretches

Bend over toe touches—Stand up straight with your hands at your sides. Keeping your legs straight, slowly bend forward at the waist while you let your hands and your head gently fall toward the floor. If you can reach the floor, place your fingers or your palms on the floor for stability. If you cannot reach the floor, place your hands on your knees or your ankles for stability. Hold for 10 seconds and then slowly return to your starting position. Repeat the exercise for 3 reps.

Bend over toe touches variation—Repeat the exercise above. While you are bent over, keep your right leg straight and bend your left leg slightly, rolling onto the ball of your left foot. Hold for 10 seconds and then straighten your left leg while you bend the right one. Hold each position for 10 seconds and then slowly return to your starting position. Repeat the exercise for 3 reps.

Bend over toe touches, legs spread apart—Stand up straight with your hands at your sides and your legs spread slightly further than shoulder width apart. Keeping your legs straight, slowly bend forward at the waist while you let your hands and your head gently fall toward the floor. If you can reach the floor, place your fingers or your palms on the floor for stability. If you cannot reach the floor, place your hands on your knees or your ankles for stability. Hold for 10 seconds and then slowly return to your starting position. Repeat the exercise for 3 reps.

You can also do these stretching exercises on the airplane if you are on a flight longer than two hours. For flights that are less than two hours, you can get up and walk up and down the aisle for ten minutes. Just make sure that you follow federal laws and remain in your seat and stay buckled up when you are supposed to and listen to the flight crew at all times. For every fifty minutes of sitting you do, you should get up and move for ten minutes. You'll stay on track with your fitness plan by using the plane time to keep yourself active.

Core on a Plane

While you are seated on the airplane, you can exercise your core with a series of simple, seated exercises that we call "Core on a Plane."

Single leg extension—Begin sitting upright in your airplane seat with your back straight, your knees bent, and your feet on the floor in front of you. Raise your right leg straight out in front of you being careful not to kick the seat. Hold for 10 seconds and then lower your right leg and repeat the exercise with your left leg. If you have longer legs and do not have the space to perform this exercise, you can place your hands on the armrests, perform a triceps extension and raise your bottom off your seat. This will give you the extra room to complete this exercise. Do 3 sets of 10 reps.

Double leg extensions—Begin sitting upright in your airplane seat with your back straight, your knees bent, and your feet on the floor in front of you. Raise both legs at the same time, straight out in front of you and hold for 10 seconds. If you have longer legs, see the single leg exercise above for a variation that will help you complete these exercises. Do 3 sets of 10 reps.

Cross over resistance—Begin sitting upright in your airplane seat with your back straight,

your knees bent, and your feet on the floor in front of you. Place the palm of your right hand on the inside of your left knee. Apply pressure with your hand onto your knee while you also raise your left knee in the direction of your right shoulder. Hold for 10 seconds and then repeat the exercise with your left hand on your right knee. This completes a repetition. Do 3 sets of 10 reps.

Same side resistance—Begin sitting upright in your airplane seat with your back straight, your knees bent, and your feet on the floor in front of you. Place the palm of your right hand on the top of your right knee. Apply pressure with your hand onto your knee while you also raise your right knee straight up in the direction of your right shoulder. Hold for 10 seconds and then repeat the exercise with your left hand on your left knee. This completes a repetition. Do 3 sets of 10 reps.

Leg squeeze in and out against resistance—Begin sitting upright in your airplane seat with your back straight, your knees bent, and your feet on the floor in front of you. Bend over slightly and place your right hand on the inside of your left knee and your left hand on the inside of your right knee. Squeeze your knees together against the resistance of your hands pushing outwards. Hold for 10 seconds. Complete 1 set of 10 repetitions.

Now place your right hand on the outside of your right knee and your left hand on the outside of your left knee. Push your legs outwards while you apply resistance with your hands pushing your knees together. Hold for 10 seconds. Complete 1 set of 10 repetitions.

ONCE YOU LAND: PREPARING TO WORK OUT ON THE ROAD

One of the most important things that you can do to ensure that you stick to your fitness plan on the road is to pack your fitness gear. To simplify your life and guarantee that you never forget anything, make a 100 Year Lifestyle ESS Kit that you keep on hand so that you can just throw it in your suitcase without any last-minute packing stress. Your ESS Kit should include:

- Workout shoes

- Workout clothes—indoor clothes or outdoor gear if you're doing endurance training outside; bring enough for every day you're away.

- Heart monitor—Make this heart monitor a second heart monitor that you always keep in your travel kit so that you are sure to have it with you while you are on the road.

- Exercise bands—If you ever get to a hotel that doesn't have a gym, your exercise bands can help you do resistance training or strength training in your room. Exercise bands are available in many different resistances so pack two or three. They are light, easy to pack, and will enhance your workouts.

- Exercise DVDs for Powercentering, yoga, Pilates, Tae Bo, kickboxing, hip hop abs, or any other workout you love

- Pedometer—you can clip this on your shoe and measure your steps when you are on the road to see how active you really are. Compare and see whether or not you take more steps on the road or when you are at home. This is another way to get a baseline of your activity level.

KEEP YOUR ROUTINE

One of the reasons that we lose our way and get off The 100 Year Lifestyle bandwagon is that when we travel our routine can get disturbed. Your awareness of this will help you to consciously choose to keep up with your routine when you are on the road. Believe it or not, this begins when you start planning your trips. Choose the times that you depart and return around your exercise routines. If you like to work out in the morning, set your schedule so you leave your departure city either in

> When you're researching your hotels, ask the reservation desk ahead of time:
>
> - Do you have a fitness center in your hotel?
>
> - What kind of equipment is in your hotel?
>
> - Is all of the equipment in working order or is any of it broken?

midmorning, afternoon, or evening so you can get your workout in before you go. If you like to work out in the afternoon or evening, do the same thing by scheduling your travel around your workouts. This might not always be possible. If you have an all-day trip, make this day a rest day and plan your workouts on the days before and after your trip.

If you get to the hotel only to find the equipment isn't actually as described, don't be afraid to confront the hotel. They are misrepresenting themselves if they give you false information. This will help the next person who wants to work out there. Also don't rely on consistency among chains. You may find that one hotel brand may have good equipment in one location and not in another. Sometimes it's more of a marketing ploy for a hotel to have a "fitness center." But more people than ever are using these fitness centers and are demanding better quality equipment.

WORK THE TIME CHANGE INTO YOUR WORKOUT

While you are on the road, if you are in a different time zone, use the time change to your advantage. If you are flying from the East Coast to the West Coast, you will probably wake up very early and have extra time in the mornings to get your workouts in. If you are flying from the West Coast to the East Coast, you will most likely stay up late and have extra time in the evenings to get your workouts in. Use the time change to your advantage when planning and keeping your workout routines.

PASS THE TEN-POUND WEIGHT PLEASE

Instead of saying pass the salt, have your business meeting in the gym or on the jogging trail. Have a business power lift instead of a business power lunch. The days of the thousand-calorie business lunch are winding down as more and more people are eating healthy. To have a power lift lunch, have your meeting while you are working out. You will be amazed at the creativity level that flows while you are moving during your meetings. Just like businesspeople like to have golf outings in an effort to get to know who they are doing business with, the same can be done during a workout together. You can have a great conversation standing side by side on the AMT or elliptical with a business associate. You can really get to know people if you are taking

Power Lift Plan

Ahead of time, ask the people you will be meeting on your trip if they work out. If they do work out, ask them if they would like to get a workout in together while you are there on business. In our training programs for doctors, we start out every meeting with a walk/talk session where we go hiking together and talk about personal development and personal growth. I have done this for corporations around the world and they love the suit-free environment where they can get real and become better people. Let's face it, happier people who feel fulfilled are also more productive employees, and in this day and age of declining employee benefits, what a great way for a company to show that they care.

a power walk or going for a run together. And spotting each other during a strength-training routine can create a level of mutual trust that can carry over into the boardroom when you get there to finalize your deals.

HEALTHY EATING ON THE ROAD

Keep the edge when it comes to your food and calorie intake while you travel. Since you'll be in different cities with unfamiliar restaurants, unfamiliar grocery stores, and an abundance of fast food options screaming in your face, maintaining the edge and planning your meals and snacks is extremely important. You can pretty much get any decent restaurant to customize your meal. Don't be afraid to ask for what you want. When you look at your menus, look for the type of foods that are listed in Chapter Four and simply ask for them. Keep in mind to choose QCs over ECs every time you are faced with a choice. Be conscious of the foods that used to be "treats" to you but are now "tricks." Say "yes" to the things that are good for you while you say "no" to the fat-creating, health-deteriorating tricks that can have loud, strong voices while you are away from home.

Being on the road can be a lonely life. Many people, when they travel, will look to fill their loneliness or that void in their soul from being away from home with food. Don't do it. Fill the hole with exercise. Fill the hole with staying in communication with the people that you love. Fill the hole with passionate work and the confidence that you gain in yourself by keeping your commitments to your ideal 100

To help you keep track of your calorie intake and your personal fitness plan on the road, use The 100 Year Lifestyle program powered by dotFIT. Visit www.100yearlifestyle.com and try it for fourteen days, free.

Year Lifestyle. But don't fill it with food.

When it comes to food on the road, draw your line in the sand and make healthy choices. If you get off track, get back on track with your next choice. Be excited and stay excited about the compelling changes you are making by committing to your 100 Year Lifestyle, not by what you are depriving yourself of by not eating the "tricks" in your history. Focus on what you will be gaining, which includes greater personal confidence, a higher level of integrity, more energy, and youthfulness—your best you.

THE HEALTHY BOTTOM LINE

Stay on schedule, stay on track, and be consistent when you are on the road. Keep the basics of your ESS routine in place. If you're supposed to work your core on any given day, work it on the road on the same schedule. If you're scheduled to do full body training, do your best to keep your routine while on the road. Obviously if you are going to work out with someone, have a creative workout day and look to incorporate some of the strategies of your workout partner or experiment with a new piece of equipment or exercise that you like. Either way keeping your fitness routine while on the road will keep you off of the weight and health roller coaster.

CHAPTER TEN:

Fitness Strategies Just for Women

Years ago a famous book made a great case that *Men Are from Mars, Women Are from Venus.* The basic premise stated that men and women are different creatures from an emotional and relationship standpoint. Well, guess what? From a workout and fitness perspective, men and women are not the same either. The obvious difference is build, but we'll get to that in a moment. A more subtle distinction that many women ignore or do not acknowledge is that by the time a woman takes care of her kids, everyone in the family's schedule, managing the household, and caring for others, she often forgets about caring for herself. While women have a higher life expectancy than men, you don't want to let your self-care slip and take your quality and quantity of life along with it.

Most women have to fit several roles into one schedule including professional, mother, caregiver, and daughter. And when someone is juggling so many things, time often slips away.

How to Get Started and Stay Engaged?

- Find a workout buddy—women are social by nature.

- Sharing fitness goals with a friend will help keep you on track because you don't want to let down your friend.

- Group fitness classes are a great start. Groups take the pressure off of the woman being in the gym.

- Find a fitness center with day care or a kid's zone.

- Exercise is great "me" time.

If a gym is just too much for you at the very beginning, you can still get started. Go for a walk to build your endurance. Take a friend, a pet, or music—or even consider heading to the mall for a walk. Once you get into it and feel better, visit a gym. Take a look around and see what's going on. Get a feel for your space and when you are ready, join.

Now, don't forget, just because you were athletic in high school or college doesn't mean you can jump back in and do what you did back then. Your body has muscle memory but you need to take it slow.

Women are big multitaskers and can usually accomplish 100 things in a day. But with such busy schedules, their fitness can sometimes fall to the bottom of the list. Guess what? If this has happened to you, it's time to move it up a bit higher and figure out a way to fit it into a busy day. How can you achieve this if all of your time is spent caring for everyone else? Well the answer is simple—find a way to create a fitness regime with reasonable goals and time limits so that you can no longer make any excuses. Don't set a lofty goal like a two-hour workout. Aim for a twenty-minute one that you know you can squeeze in.

Corry Matthews, who has a master's degree in sports medicine and is a member of the Gold's Gym Fitness Institute, says women have a common concern about finding time, but she says time shouldn't be the reason you don't work out at all. Women out there might want to have five hours per week to work out, but that goal might not be totally realistic. So Corry says any time you can devote in a week can become your fitness program. Whatever time you have available—twenty minutes, one hour—you can create a program to get you moving, as long as you follow it.

Women should take care of themselves, and they will have less stress or even a stress-free life if they do. So get started!

DON'T BE INTIMIDATED!

First of all, if you're starting a fitness regime, remember that you're not alone. The gym is probably full of women who feel some level of anxiety about working out. Women also often feel like they can't get started until they lose weight or look better. Get over that fast. Put on some sweats and get in there and have fun. The results you achieve will inspire you to keep going. Don't let movie stars and magazine pictures psyche you out—that's not how real women look.

And don't let your age talk you out of joining a gym either. There are so many qualified trainers out there who can accommodate aging women—even beginners. A trainer will help prevent injuries and make sure you keep coming in and feel confident. Personal trainers are there to show you step by step how to succeed and avoid injury.

If you're really nervous, grab a girlfriend to get in there with you. And get your ESS in

Tips on Finding a Personal Trainer

- Interview trainers like it's a job interview.
- Decide if you feel more comfortable with a man or a woman.
- Ask specific questions at the front desk.
- Switch trainers: Most trainers will not be offended if you don't think they are working for you to get the results you want.

Why should women do strength training?

- To gain energy and confidence

- To increase metabolism

- To increase lean body mass

- It reduces their risk for osteoporosis.

- It's beneficial for the heart. It's a muscle like the rest of the muscles.

- To improve their immune system

- To stay healthier longer

shape together. Join a women-only gym if that helps or find a female trainer.

A DIFFERENT BUILD

The second major difference in fitness between men and women is pretty basic: Women are built differently. Different bodies, different challenges, and different strengths and limitations are all reasons women need to vary their workout to a certain degree. One thing that does remain the same, however, is the need to focus on getting your ESS in shape. That standard applies to men, women, and children of all ages. Here's how the ESS applies to women:

Endurance—Heart disease is the number one killer of women, so the American Heart Association recommends thirty minutes of cardiovascular activity a day. But if you can aim for an hour a day, you can work all of the ESS elements into your workout.

Structure is extremely important for women. Women's joints are different from

men's, so it's necessary to follow proper form during your workouts—especially if less time is spent doing it. Proper alignment will ensure better results. Corry has found that when her clients are aligned and balanced, they get better results because their muscles and nerves are working properly. If you are a beginner to exercise, she recommends a spinal screening.

Strength—Elaborate weight training is not necessary for women. The ESS sequences in this book are a great start and give women a lot of flexibility. One of the main physical differences between men and women lies in the pelvic girdle for women, where they are built for childbirth. When it comes to strength, women have stronger lower bodies, and men have stronger upper bodies.

WORKOUT GEAR FOR WOMEN

Also remember, women require some gear specific only to their gender. Getting the right gear, especially chest support, is critical to maximize both the enjoyment and impact of your workout routine. If you're top heavy wear supportive clothing. Find a good sports bra, and leave vanity out of the equation. You need to worry about your back. You want to make sure you wear the right shoes, too, so you don't injure yourself, especially when you're starting out. Feet are your foundation, especially if you want to avoid shin splints and spinal problems. Custom-made Spinal Pelvic Stabilizers that you insert in your shoes can make a remarkable difference.

FEMALE FRIENDLY WORKOUT

Women may want to do elaborate exercises to get their lower body in shape, but lunges are a

ESS Story: Shele Hauser

I was a hairstylist and a gymnastic coach for many years, and I trained upper level gymnasts. They were my life, and my kids, since I would spend over thirty hours a week with them. I was fit and healthy; I had great endurance and a gymnast's strength. Then one day when I was spotting a gymnast I felt a sharp shooting pain go down my arm and into my hand. I could not move it without having pain. It was constant pain, and I could put my finger on where it hurt. I would try to hold a bowl of cereal in my hand, and I would almost drop it because of the sharp pain. I couldn't work either job. I had been out of balance and didn't know it until the final straw broke the camel's back.

I went to see an orthopedic surgeon, and I had some tests done. I had two surgeries and I did rehab, but my arm was much worse than before. I cried a lot. My range of motion had gotten worse also. I was so frustrated! I could not do anything. I complained to the doctor, and he told me that the elbow was a tricky part of the body, and difficult to work on. I tried one more doctor and one more surgery. In over two and a half years, I had three surgeries, and I could still only use one arm. I needed help with everything—even the simplest task of opening a can of soup. I had to wear pull-on clothes. It was very frustrating for me not to be active.

After the third surgery, the surgeon told me the elbow was tricky, and that I would have to live with the pain the rest of my life and take Advil a couple times a day. I would have to find a job that wouldn't use my upper extremities. Immediately, I was thinking of the kids that I have trained for years, as tears ran down my face. What was

woman's best friend. They can help your entire lower body get in shape quickly and easily.

You can try any of the following:

- **Stepping Forward Lunges**—Begin by standing straight with your feet together. Take a giant step forward with your right leg only. Let your left foot curl up onto the ball of your foot while your left knee approaches a few inches from the floor. Bring your right leg back to its original position and stand up straight again. Now repeat this lunge stepping forward with your left leg.

I going to do? I loved styling peoples' hair also. I would have to quit both jobs and deal with the pain I still had. I also worried I might never be able to pick up and hold my baby in my arms or play with my kids the way I would like to as a healthy person would.

I had to deal with this pain in my arm for over five years. It was one of the worst times in my life. This finally changed when I went to a chiropractic school clinic, and I had a complete structure examination done. My husband asked the doctor if he could look at my arm. What did I have to lose, so I let him examine it, and I showed him where it hurt. I had him adjust it, and it hurt for a little while after, but I had immediate improvement with my range of motion, and my pain was less. I couldn't believe it. This changed my life! I have no pain, and I have full range of motion back in my arm.

I was able to go back to coaching gymnastics, and I went back to styling hair, something that I was told I would never do again. I was thrilled with the improvements I was making.

A year later, I got pregnant. I had chiropractic care, with Dr. Greg Hauser in Phoenix, Arizona, throughout my pregnancy. I had a natural childbirth with no drugs, and I was able to hold my baby boy with no pain. What great joy I have to be able to be the mom I always wanted to be. Chiropractic care has changed my life for the better. And because of that, I have been off all medication for ten years, and I have no pain in my arm at all! I have been headache free, and I do not get strep throat anymore. Living to 100 doesn't seem scary anymore. I am excited about getting there in style and enjoying the journey along the way.

- **Stepping Backwards Lunges**—Begin by standing straight with your feet together. Take a giant step backwards with your right leg only. Keep your left foot on the ground while your right knee approaches a few inches from the floor. Bring your right leg back to its original position and stand up straight again. Now repeat this lunge stepping backwards with your left leg.

How can you achieve a lean look? Do higher reps, with lower weight.

3–4 sets of 12–20 reps

How can you build strength? Lower reps, with higher weight.

1–2 sets of 8–12 reps

The most difficult lunge requires ten minutes of stepping, walking lunges. This can be done by doing the Stepping Forward Lunges above, except instead of coming back to your original position, you can alternate lunging forward with one foot after the other. Make it even more challenging by holding onto weights in each hand.

Squats are also a universal strength exercise for women that work across all age groups from the young to seniors. This exercise creates pelvic strength during childbearing years and during your senior years. Squats boost your strength and make sure you'll always be able to lift yourself up as you age. Seniors should modify the squat by sitting and standing from a chair with no hands so that they protect their hip joints. Pregnant women need to make sure their squats are supported so that they remain balanced. When performing squats always be sure to watch your knees—they shouldn't extend too far over your toes and your knee should be hinging not twisting.

Women and Working Out

Myth: Women shouldn't do strength training because they'll bulk up and look manly.

Fact: Women are biologically different than men and they don't build muscle or lose weight as quickly as men. Here are a few of the benefits women will get from strength training.

- Women should do some strength training to build long lean muscles and boost their metabolism.

- Women need to do intense workouts with weights, but do more reps, with lighter weights, and exercise at a quicker pace than men do to achieve a higher rate of calorie burning.

- Strength training will lessen joint injuries and help provide healthier, injury-free participation in recreational sports.

EXERCISE THAT REFLECTS A WOMAN'S LIFE

Women should make sure to focus on their core, because everyday life requires strength around the middle. Getting kids or grandchildren in and out of car seats is an example of a movement that requires twisting awkward movements, so you want to do specific exercises that mimic and strengthen the core. Spend a lot of time with the core crazy exercises in this book or try Pilates or yoga.

NUTRITION AND EXERCISE

Food and exercise go hand in hand when you're trying to get in shape, but many women make a big mistake. They eat too little. Don't make that mistake. You need to eat enough to fuel your body properly. The one thing you must avoid is getting into starvation mode. If you starve yourself, your body goes into a survival mode and holds onto the fat. The body becomes very efficient at holding on to weight. It's important to eat properly if you're in your reproductive years because food supports healthy lactation. Create your customized meal plan at www.100yearlifestyle.com.

PREGNANCY AND EXERCISE

All the things we just discussed are critical to remember for all women, but if you're pregnant, you'll want to make sure you make some modifications throughout the pregnancy to keep you and your baby healthy. Corry, who just gave birth to her first child, makes the following important suggestions, but make sure you talk to your doctor about your exercise routine and get the okay to continue or get started.

The following workout and diet modifications for prenatal women cover each trimester.

First Trimester Exercise

- Keep heart rate under 140 beats per minute to prevent overheating.

- If you are currently exercising, ask your doctor about maintaining a similar training routine.

- If you're new to exercise, find a trainer.

- If you find you tire easily, it is probably due to baby development. Listen to your body.

- Prenatal yoga is great for someone who has never exercised much. Pilates is fine, too.

- Endorphins can negate morning sickness so exercise will help.

First Trimester Eating

- Eat 200–300 additional calories a day.

- Make healthy food choices.

- Choose whole grain carbohydrates, fruits, veggies, and lowfat proteins.

- Graze by eating five or six small meals per day to stabilize your blood glucose level.

Second Trimester Exercise

- During this period your entire structure and center of gravity changes. The baby moves up into the abdomen.

- For endurance, explore low impact options.

- Avoid lying on your back!

- Yoga and swimming are great for endurance.

- Any weight training must be supported with good posture and structural alignment.

- Listen to your body.

Second Trimester Eating

- Eat 200–300 additional calories a day.

- Make healthy choices.

- Choose whole grain carbohydrates, fruits, veggies, and lowfat proteins.

- Graze by eating five or six small meals for blood glucose level.

- Listen to your body.

- Maintain great communication with your doctor and/or midwife, and follow their recommendations.

Third Trimester Exercises

- Avoid lying on your back!

- Thirty minutes of moderate exercise throughout your pregnancy is fine.

- Do not exercise more than two hours when pregnant.

- All exercise must be supported.

- Continue to eat five or six small meals throughout the day

- Listen to your body.

- Follow your doctor and/or midwife's recommendations.

PREGNANCY AND STRUCTURE

Exercise can be an important part of a healthy pregnancy, and getting and keeping your ESS in shape can make a big difference for you. When I was in practice, I loved taking care of pregnant women and their families. Chiropractic adjustments can give women tremendous pain relief, eliminate stress, and make your pregnancy much more enjoyable. There are a variety of chiropractic techniques that can be great for your spinal and pelvic alignment that can be utilized right up to the day of delivery. Many obstetricians refer patients to chiropractors for this and many other healthy reasons. Many of the chiropractors listed at www.100yearlifestyle .com have taken certification and continuing education courses and specialize in the care of pregnant women and newborn babies. Visit the Web site and see if there is a provider near you. Ask them if they have experience working with pregnancy and newborns. Keeping your structure aligned and balanced, with the nerves working properly, can make your nine months much more enjoyable.

If you are a higher-risk pregnancy, make sure you discuss a fitness plan with your OB/GYN and follow their recommendations completely.

AFTER DELIVERY WORKOUT REGIME

If you're ready to get back to the gym after giving birth, just make sure you take it slowly. Ask your doctor when you can begin your workouts again. For most women, waiting a full two weeks after natural delivery is recommended, and you should begin slowly. If you've had a C-section, you'll need more time.

Many women can resume their workouts within six to eight weeks after delivery, as long as they've received clearance from their doctor. You can start backwards doing the third trimester exercises first, then second trimester, and finally first trimester exercises. You may need to take your time and take six months to get back to first trimester workouts.

Otherwise, at three to four months if you're feeling up to it, you can resume your pre-pregnancy routine. Take care of your core and your structure and then add strength training, doing small exercises for limbs. To start to boost your endurance, try endurance exercises like walking when you walk the baby carrier or push the stroller. For structure a back or front carrier is better than a sling-type carrier.

Just make sure you make time to heal the body through getting your ESS in shape and you will enjoy a healthier life. And don't forget to get and keep your spine in line to help your body bounce back from delivery or surgery.

Remember that exercise not only makes you feel better, but it can help you heal faster and might actually boost the joy you get from motherhood.

CARETAKER TAKE CARE

If you have not been taking care of yourself, it is time to get back on track. Women live longer than men because they tend to be more committed to their own self-care. They are more likely to be proactive when it comes to their health and they make it a priority. They are more likely to exercise, they are more likely to make regular visits to their chiropractor, and they are more likely to go for preventative health care checkups. Now, through The 100 Year Lifestyle Workout, you can take this balanced approach to fitness to ensure that as you age, you keep your body in the best shape possible.

If you are like many women who take care of your family, including your children and grandchildren, as well as maybe even your parents and grandparents, it is important to take care of yourself. You will be better able to take care of your loved ones if you are healthy and strong.

Don't wait for a crisis. Make quality of life your motivating factor and get in the best shape of your life, regardless of your age.

CHAPTER ELEVEN:

Fitness in Your Fifties, Sixties, and Beyond

If you're over 60 and you're reading this book, it's not too late to live The 100 Year Lifestyle and get your ESS in shape. In fact, it's more important than ever. It's no secret that our bodies change as we age. Some changes are obvious, while others are more subtle. Many people age gracefully and remain active, alert, and vibrant throughout their extended lives. Their physiologic age may be quite a bit younger than their chronological age. Others may experience the effects of osteoporosis and osteoarthritis, which can gradually diminish their abilities to participate fully in activities. Knowing what to expect and taking steps to counterbalance the effects of aging can help you maintain a young spirit and an independent life, even if you are getting started when you are in your sixties. Getting and keeping your ESS in shape can help delay the onset and slow the progression of many age-related changes.

Before we get started on some 100 Year Lifestyle Workout strategies, let's revisit the disclaimer. Make an appointment with your cardiologist and have your heart examined, and make an appointment with your chiropractor to check out your spine. Also, revisit the sixteen avoidable mistakes and make sure you start out on the right track to build momentum with your plan and prevent any mishaps from setting you back. It is also important to understand what can happen to your body if you don't keep yourself fit, and how your body can reverse the effects of aging through fitness.

HOW AGING CAN AFFECT YOUR BODY

Physiological aging refers to the changes in structure and functioning of the body that occur over a life span. Many of these changes are involuntary and take place very gradually while others occur over a short period. If we can better understand the effects aging has on the tissues and systems of the body, we can modify lifestyle changes to counteract the effects of aging. Changes that may occur in the cardiovascular system include a decrease in the elasticity of the blood vessels and heart valves, restricted blood flow due to the thickening of the vessel walls and because of the fatty deposits lining the blood vessels, and a decrease in the ability of the heart to pump out as much blood with each beat. As a result you may feel fatigued, become short of breath more easily, and have less capacity for physical exertion.

Decreased elasticity of the lungs may also occur with aging. This may affect your lungs' ability to utilize oxygen, as well as your ability to cough and take deep breaths. You may be more prone to fatigue and shortness of breath on exertion and become more susceptible to infections. As we age there may be a gradual loss of muscle tone, elasticity, and strength. But what is more significant is that your endurance or strength to perform certain tasks may also diminish. The skeletal system gradually changes over the years and can become porous and brittle, as the bones lose calcium as well as their density. This may be more pronounced in women. As a result, you may become more prone to fractures, notice a decrease in height, or even develop a stoop in your posture.

It is not uncommon to experience a gradual decline in the activity of the thyroid gland, as well as decline in the ability of the pancreas to produce insulin. As a result, the body has more trouble using fats and sugars and converting them into energy. You may note an increase in weight and an increased blood sugar level when you visit the doctor, who may tell you that you have adult onset diabetes. You may find you have less energy or ability to handle stress.

The digestive tract is a resilient system, but some changes can occur as we age that may cause distress. There is a gradual slowing of the system as well as a decrease in the secretion of saliva and enzymes that are necessary for digestion. As a result, there may be problems with indigestion, elimination, and adequate absorption of nutrients.

Aging also affects our nervous system. The messages take a slightly longer time to pass from the nerves to the muscles, and the muscles take a slightly longer time to react to these messages. Also, there may be a decrease in the perception of pain and an increase in the time to react to it.

A HEALTHY LIFESTYLE = SUCCESSFUL AGING

The U.S. Department of Health and Human Services and the CDC report successful aging is largely determined by individual lifestyle choices and not by genetic inheritance. If you do not modify your lifestyle, many of these physiological effects of aging can degenerate into chronic conditions such as heart disease, hypertension, arthritis, diabetes, and osteoporosis. This can result in unnecessary lost quality of life for you, and for millions of others, and lead to premature death and a significant financial burden on our health care system. The treatment and management of chronic conditions make up 76 percent of U.S. medical costs while $161.3 billion is lost to the economy. A growing body of research suggests that much of the decline attributed to aging actually comes from being sedentary, and that regular exercise can help people remain healthy and independent as they get older.

In spite of the volumes of evidence regarding the health benefits of regular exercise, the U.S. Department of Health and Human Services reports that one third of people sixty-five and over are sedentary; 54 percent of men and 66 percent of women over age seventy-five get no physical activity at all. The National Health Interview Survey goes on to say that only 11 percent of older adults meet strength training recommendations. The costs in dollars and in lives due to physical inactivity are staggering. Dr. Teresa Keenan, senior research advisor for AARP, estimates that physical inactivity causes more than 300,000 deaths and $77 billion in direct health care costs each year. According to statistics reported by the President's Council on Physical Fitness and Sports (PCPFS), physical inactivity accounts for 15 percent of the U.S. $1.4 trillion health care budget: $298 billion on the treatment of cardiovascular disease, $98 billion on type 2 diabetes, and $8 billion on arthritis.

Unfortunately it is predominately the senior population that suffers from these chronic conditions. The PCPFS reports that 88 percent of the elderly suffer from chronic conditions, and 23 percent of all deaths are caused by major chronic diseases, according to the U.S. Department of Health and Human Services. When we see that there are presently forty-six million people in this country over the age of sixty, and with these numbers rising to seventy-six million over the next fifteen years due to the exploding aging Baby Boomer population, how can we find a solution to the financial crisis in our health care system when statistics from the CDC state that one third of all U.S. health care costs are spent on adults sixty-five years and older, and Medicare alone spends $84 billion per year on five major chronic conditions?

To preempt a continued decline in the health of our society and the unsustainable rising costs of our health care system, we must collectively choose to move and *get our ESS in shape*! The father of modern medicine, Hippocrates, in his later years valued exercise, prescribing it for mental as well as physical illness. In his writings *Regimen in Health*, he wrote:

Eating alone will not keep a man well; he must also take exercise. Food and exercise, while possessing opposite qualities yet work together to produce health . . . And it is necessary . . . to discern the power of various exercises, both natural exercises and artificial, to know which to them tends to increase flesh and which to lessen it; and not only this but also to proportion exercise to bulk of food, to the constitution of the patient, to the age of the individual.

Exercise should be many and of all kinds, running on the double track increased gradually. Sharp walks after exercise, short walks in the sun after dinner, many walks in the early morning quiet to begin with, increasing till they are violent and then gently finishing.

Hippocrates was an advocate of exercise and an advocate of a healthy spine. His writings described the importance of addressing all three components of the ESS model in The 100 Year Lifestyle Workout, and we should take his advice. Chiropractic organizations have long written and spoken about the benefits of exercise and a healthy spine. Medical organizations are now recognizing the need to promote the health benefits of exercise. A recent report by the College of Chest Physicians stated that exercise capacity is inversely associated with health care costs, and concluded that a preponderance of evidence clearly points to the potential for improvement in both the physical and economic health of our society that can be achieved through improving physical fitness. A joint venture between the AMA and the American College of Sports Medicine titled *Exercise is Medicine* is an initiative that directs all medical providers to treat exercise as a vital sign and to discuss and recommend exercise to all of their patients. They encourage the medical profession to work closely with other health care providers and the fitness industry to improve the physical activity level of our nation. Even the prestigious *Journal of the American Medical Association* states that the practice of regular exercise along with a Mediterranean diet, moderate alcohol consumption, and not smoking can decrease the risk of death over the next ten years by 50 percent.

When asked why older adults should exercise, National Institute on Aging director Dr. Richard J. Hodes responded:

It's much more than okay for older people to exercise. And importantly, that is a conviction that is based not just on intuition but as a result of a good deal of research over the past years. It was judged that exercise was too dangerous, too vigorous and that older people, because of frailty, were more likely to be injured or damaged by exercise. However, a number of well-conducted, controlled studies have shown that a variety of exercises are not only safe for older people but have enormous advantage. This includes aerobic exercise, endurance training, that is good for conditioning of heart and lungs as well as rather vigorous weight training, strength training, which has shown the ability in

people in their sixties, seventies, eighties, and even nineties, to significantly increase muscle mass, most importantly, muscle strength, and most importantly of all, to translate that increase of strength into the ability to carry out functions of daily living; to climb stairs, to shop, to carry packages. These are things that are important to maintaining independence and health throughout the life span.

Exercise is an essential part of living a healthy life, and also a healthy long life. Living to 100 is a marathon and not a sprint, so the training for your longevity should be a part of your lifestyle at every age.

Many governmental organizations understand the importance of physical activity. The PCPFS recommends that the promotion of a physically active lifestyle should occur through the inclusion of physical activity at social gatherings. Seniors should be allowed free access to strength-training equipment and recreational facilities, and should be educated on the consequences of a sedentary lifestyle on their vitality, quality of life, and ability to perform the tasks of daily living. The Division of Aging and Seniors states that regular enjoyable exercise is currently the most significant route to better health and is a more straightforward and economical means to lifelong health than medication and acute care. In light of the strength of the evidence on the benefits of physical activity, the focus of future action resides mainly in the identification and implementation of successful interventions for older adults.

ESS Story: Annette Cullers

In addition to being blessed with excellent genes, I also had parents who introduced my siblings and me to a very active way of life, and we have been living the principles of The 100 Year Lifestyle. They stressed how and when to choose healthy foods, especially avoiding an excess of sweets and fats. Swimming, tennis, and basketball were my favorite sports. I was swimming and diving before I was three years old, which is something all parents should do for their children. That was the basics of my healthy bone structure and one of the three "ESS" that guides the way to better and healthier living. The endurance I got through a lifetime in sports provided the development of great strength that I maintained throughout my life.

In any town I was in, I always found a good gym and would often help trainers teach young and older people how to become more active and encourage daily exercise programs. People are amazed when they see me exercising at the gym I belong to in nearby Winchester, Virginia. They try to guess my age, and usually they guess about twenty to twenty-five years lower than my correct age of ninety-three years. That, of course, is nice to hear.

My life is focused on keeping a good posture, maintaining flexibility, and having a healthy daily diet of plenty of raw vegetables, few meats, and not too many sweets. I have an occasional glass of wine or an alcoholic drink. I was often teased or ridiculed by my peers in the 1950s and 60s for

GETTING YOUR ESS IN SHAPE CAN REVERSE THE EFFECTS OF AGING

According to the American College of Sports Medicine (ACSM), by the year 2030 the number of individuals in the U.S. sixty years and older will reach seventy million and people eighty-five years and older will be the fastest-growing segment of the population. But whatever your age, exercise can help. Endurance decreases as we age. In a classic study of walking and mortality in seven hundred men enrolled in the Honolulu Heart Program, the mortality rate among the men who walked less than one mile per day was nearly twice that among those who walked more than two miles per day (studies of women show equally potent results).

not smoking or drinking at lunch as most did in those days. Seeing too many of my cohorts in the national press in Washington go down the sliding path to being alcoholics and losing their jobs was enough to convince me not to do the same.

My mother was smart enough to have a chiropractor visit our home in the little town of Cordele, Georgia, about two or three times a month to align the spines of her four children—a practice I continued throughout my long life. I exercise morning and night for about thirty minutes. I visit my chiropractor, Dr. Joe Cheff in Woodstock, Virginia, at least twice a month, though in the past year because of a botched knee operation, the visits had to be more frequent. I quickly learned from him what I was doing wrong in my twice daily exercise program, how to handle strengthening my body, and how to chart my endurance habits in sports.

Endure and be patient— giving your body time to respond to exercise is of paramount importance. Get on the scale every morning—without fail—and, if you have gained an ounce, watch your calorie intake for a day or so until you are back to the desired weight.

Should I ever make the mistake of not following the ESS principles of The 100 Year Lifestyle, I can quickly tell the difference in my body, my lifestyle, and my attitude. I have been lucky to have always been an upbeat person and I see the water glass of life filled and brimming with promise even at ninety-three years young.

In another equally impressive study, data collected on more than 41,000 men and women from 1990 to 2001 was analyzed to find the relationship between walking and mortality. It was reported that men and women who walked thirty minutes or more per day during the study period had fewer deaths than those who walked less than thirty minutes.

Strength and muscle mass can increase at any age in response to exercise. In an important study of weightlifting and older adults conducted with 100 male and female residents of a nursing home in Boston (age range: seventy-two to ninety-eight, average age eighty-seven), subjects lifted weights with their legs two times a week for ten weeks. At the end of the study, there was an increase in thigh mass of 2.7 percent, walking speed increased 12 percent, and leg strength increased a whopping 113 percent!

Structure and bone density tend to decrease as we age, which can lead to osteoporosis and increased risk of fracture. In two different studies of weightlifting, one of middle-aged and older men (fifty to seventy years old) who lifted weights three times a week for sixteen weeks, and the other of women forty to seventy years of age who lifted twice a week for one year, bone density in the legs and backs of subjects in both studies increased.

One of the most exciting areas of exercise research is the investigation of cognitive function. In a study where researchers used an MRI machine to measure the amount of brain tissue in adults fifty-five years of age and older, they found, consistent with other studies of aging and brain volume, that there were substantial declines in brain tissue density as a function of age in areas of the brain responsible for thinking and memory. The losses in these areas, however, were substantially reduced as a function of cardiovascular fitness. In other words, the fittest individuals had the most brain tissue.

FITNESS GOALS IF YOU'RE OVER SIXTY

If you are over sixty and you want to stay active and healthy for the remaining decades of your life, you must get and keep your ESS in shape. So the question becomes, how much exercise do I need for health and fitness if I am over sixty? The ACSM and American Heart Association recommend a combination of four types of exercise for older adults to achieve maximum health and vitality. Older adults need moderate-intensity endurance training for a minimum of thirty minutes, five days each week or vigorous-intensity endurance training for a minimum of twenty minutes three days each week.

To maintain health and physical independence, older adults will benefit from performing activities that maintain or increase muscular strength and endurance for a minimum of two days each week. It is recommended that eight to ten exercises be performed on two or more nonconsecutive days per week using the major muscle groups. To maintain the flexibility necessary for regular physical activity and daily life, older adults should perform activities that maintain or increase flexibility at least two days each week for at least ten minutes each day. To reduce risk of injury from falls, older adults with substantial risk of falls should perform exercises that maintain or improve balance.

There's no need to try and make up for years of inactivity overnight. In fact, there are excellent opportunities for seniors to exercise and get their ESS in shape. Start slowly and build up gradually. If that means starting with just five minutes of walking, then that's what you ought to do. In fact, one of my favorite plans to recommend for getting started is the five-minutes-out, five-minutes-back plan. You walk out for five minutes, turn around, and walk back. One of the best ways to get motivated and stay that way is to set goals. Be as specific and realistic as possible, and remember that it's not how much you do when you get started but that you simply get started.

Walking, dancing, biking, and swimming are all good options for aerobic exercise to build your endurance. Wear a heart monitor or a pedometer to measure your progress. Also check out your local senior center, recreation center, Y, or local fitness center for classes that are appropriate for you. You don't need to pump iron in a gym to do resistance training that builds your strength. If you prefer to exercise at home, I recommend exercise tubing if you're looking for a simple but effective way to do resistance exercise. This tubing looks like a rubber hose and can be purchased with a variety of resistances depending on your current level of strength. Exercise tubing is an inexpensive and versatile way to begin a strength-training routine.

There are lots of good resources for stretching exercises. Yoga is great if you want to learn how to stretch, or you may find stretching classes at your local recreation center or senior center. Stretching classes are a great way to relax, improve your flexibility, and maybe even meet some new people. You can perform a simple exercise to improve balance by holding on to a sturdy chair for balance and lifting your right knee up toward your chest, then lowering it to your starting position. You can bend your left knee slightly. Repeat 10–15 times with the right leg; then do the left leg. You can progress to touching the chair with one finger for balance, then eventually not holding it at all, and finally with your eyes closed. You can also try alternating the marching between left and right leg instead of one set with one leg.

A unique, state of the art program that combines Endurance, Strength, and Structure training into one thirty-minute workout that will definitely get your ESS in shape is the Stay Fit Seniors circuit training system. This growing senior-specific wellness program is being delivered around the country in doctors' offices and is referred to by Jack LaLanne as the "perfect thirty-minute workout that can save peoples' lives." Seniors work out in a circuit-training format, alternating resistance training on state of the art hydraulic exercise equipment and cardio-walk-in-place stations where you learn about health and nutrition on flat screen TVs while listening to oldies music.

Dr. Anthony Lauro has a Stay Fit Seniors center attached to his chiropractic practice in Pomona, New York. In a recent interview Dr. Lauro said: "I love seeing my senior patients embracing their lives. They get their adjustments, they get a great workout in, and they go back into their life as healthy, energetic young people. This is the way that aging should be." This seniors-only environment and simple to use system promotes physical, mental, and social well-being and exemplifies the ESS principles of The 100 Year Lifestyle Workout and all the other elements of The 100 Year Lifestyle as well.

YOU CAN BREAK RECORDS AT ANY AGE

There have been many people throughout history who have made some of their greatest accomplishments well into the later years of their lives. Benjamin Franklin only retired from public service when he was eighty-two years old. Susan B. Anthony was past eighty when she formed the International Woman Suffrage

Alliance. George Bernard Shaw was working on his last play, *Why She Would Not*, when he was ninety-four. Robert Frost was eighty-eight when his last volume of poems, *In the Clearing*, was published. Winston Churchill was seventy-nine when he received the Nobel Prize for literature. Pablo Picasso produced 347 engravings in his eighty-seventh year.

More recently, at age seventy, fitness icon Jack LaLanne swam a mile and a half off Long Beach Harbor pulling seventy boats with seventy people, while handcuffed. Long rider Gene Glasscock at age seventy completed a horseback journey of over twenty thousand miles and three years in his quest to visit every state capital in the lower forty-eight states. He is raising scholarship money for the children of Paraguay and sending a message to senior citizens.

At age sixty Steve Fossett became the first person to fly around the world alone without stopping or re-fueling, and during his tragically shortened life set a number of records in the air, on water, and on land, Bill Anderson, a seventy-eight-year-old bicycler, completed his ride from San Diego, California, to Jacksonville Beach, Florida, and received a police escort as he completed the three thousand mile trip and raised over $3,000 for the homeless.

George Brunstad, who is the uncle of movie star Matt Damon, became the oldest person to swim the English Channel and raised at least $11,000 for an orphanage in Haiti at the same time. He completed the fete after celebrating his seventieth birthday. Lucille Borgen of Babson Park, Florida, amazed the crowd at the sixty-second annual Water Ski National Championships by winning the Women 10 slalom and tricks event on her ninety-first birthday. She is the oldest competitor to ever ski at the Nationals. We should hold these people and their accomplishments as an example that life doesn't have to diminish with age.

Embrace your longevity, no matter what your age. If you are just getting started, adopt this fitness plan. If you are already fit, enroll in the Senior Olympics and challenge your body and mind. Embrace your ideal 100 Year Lifestyle. Start your life fresh today with decades of experience under your belt and you will realize that your best is yet to come.

CHAPTER TWELVE:

Setting Up a Home Gym: Living the Lifestyle at Home

There's a great way to get your ESS in shape that leaves no room for excuses: Set up a home gym. A home gym can be as simple as finding a small amount of space on your living room floor to a fully equipped room with the latest and greatest equipment. You can do the core, endurance, strength, and structure exercises within the book from the comfort of home. And you've taken the drive time out of the equation if you're trying to squeeze a workout into a busy schedule.

Nothing is more convenient than a home gym, especially if you work at home. You can get up in the morning and start your day with a great workout, jump in the shower, and walk into your home office and start your work day. You can even save your shower for later in the day and stay in your workout clothes if you don't have a meeting. Having a personally customized home gym can increase your focus and productivity when you work at home.

You're striving for three things with your home gym: consistency, enjoyment, and results, because the convenience comes with the territory. In order to achieve all three, the set-up is important. You can do this in a couple of ways depending on your space and the amount of money you want to spend. We'll give you two

examples of home gym options—one is inexpensive and portable, and one is more permanent, requires more space, and will cost you a little more money. Either way, your investment in a home gym will be well worth it and provide you with a convenient, enjoyable 100 Year Lifestyle fitness solution.

Make sure the space you're using is designated as your space to work out, regardless of which approach you take. Make it a place you feel passionately about and that you enjoy being in. Even if you're doing a small, inexpensive version with portable equipment, create a space you really like and actually want to go to each day. And don't make it double duty space that can be stressful, like the kids' toy room. Make it a workout space that's special to you.

QUICK INEXPENSIVE HOME GYM

Choose the space and designate it as your area within which to exercise. It can be the living room, the bedroom, or the basement, but pick a spot to call yours. Set up a DVD player and a TV in a convenient spot so that you can watch the tube if you want to, or use a DVD to work out with. Once you choose your equipment— dumbbells, exercise balls, bands, or yoga mats—bundle them up into a box or basket and park them in the corner of your designated space. Have a plan to move the furniture so you know what you need to move in order to easily begin your workout, start breaking a sweat, and then quickly and easily put things away. You want this process to be as quick and easy as possible.

Leave yourself enough space to move—three or four feet more than your body when your arms and legs are extended. If for example you're six feet tall, carve out a nine by nine foot space for yourself especially if you're doing some dynamic stretching.

Also make sure you put a mat down so that when you sweat you minimize the wear and tear on your floor or carpet.

HIGHER-END HOME FITNESS

For those of you who really want to take your home fitness to another level, you can install a first-class home gym. You can fill it with top of the line endurance equipment like a bike or elliptical machine, and you can have some strength machines as well to round out your workout. There's enough high-quality equipment out there available for home purchase that you can make your home gym as effective a tool for getting in shape as a gym membership. You might still want to call on the help of a personal trainer if you're just getting started. Maybe start with a trainer in a gym before you make your purchase to see exactly what kind of equipment is best for you to use depending on your fitness level. Do your homework; talk to the pros and buy quality stuff because you want to be able to include all of the elements of your ESS workout in your home equipment. Who knows, it may even become the place your friends drop by to do their workouts as well! They may like your space better than the one they've been paying for at the local club.

When I was designing my home gym, I went to Precor's Web site at www.precor.com. They have a space planner that helped me lay out my exact home gym, based on the equipment that I wanted to purchase. The program takes into account the doors and windows for optimal set-up. This made the process easy and

Ask the Pros

Annie Beason, Precor Home Gym Equipment Expert says:

- Getting equipment into your home is the start of a commitment.

- Speak with a fitness professional and explain any injuries that you have, and get equipment that can be adjusted to fit your size as well as compensate for those injuries.

- At a minimum, get one piece of equipment for endurance and one piece for strength. You can always add more to your home gym as time goes on.

helped to ensure that the equipment fit properly in the room. Can you imagine how much money you would waste if you didn't go through this process? Today, most fitness stores and manufacturers will help you lay out your home gym for optimal space utilization and function. You should definitely take advantage of this service.

WHAT IS FUNCTIONAL TRAINING EQUIPMENT?

Functional training equipment, like the 323 from Precor, is workout equipment that mirrors movements you'd make in your daily routine or favorite sports. Its exercises cross multiple platforms of movement—mimicking things you'll do all day long outside of the gym. Functional equipment allows you to mix up your workout and build strength in different areas of the body to provide you with a complete all-over workout. If you're at a higher performance level, you can use functional equipment to boost your sports-specific training areas.

Functional machines give you an endless number of exercises—more room for creativity and growth as your fitness level grows. You can choose to stabilize yourself on a bench or a stability ball and work on your core while you strengthen the rest of your body. You can customize a routine to help your golf game, tennis game, or soccer or basketball skills. Because the movements are user defined, the options are limitless.

MACHINE-DEFINED EQUIPMENT

Machine-defined pieces of equipment are more limiting, with six or so different exercises you can do, and you might eventually outgrow or

Finding the Best Equipment for Your Space

For Endurance Training:
Larger Space (7 x 3): Elliptical or Treadmill
Smaller Space (5 x 2): Bike or Climber

For Strength Training:
Functional equipment (with cables, like the 323 from Precor)
Free weights system or specific machine-defined equipment
An all-in one functional piece might take up less space.

get tired of them. For example you might buy a piece that only works your biceps. That's not to say this piece isn't a great investment, but if you're trying to maximize your space at home, then you might want something more broad based and flexible in its use for your workout. The typical machine-defined home gym has exercises for chest, back, shoulders, biceps, triceps, quadriceps, and hamstrings, isolating those muscle groups alone during the workout. On the other hand, functional training equipment allows you to incorporate secondary and tertiary supportive muscle groups, which is more applicable in real life.

WHAT TO WATCH FOR WHEN YOU PURCHASE EQUIPMENT

Folding equipment works well if you have space limitations, because it saves room and you can put it away, but out of sight means out of mind, too. Are you sure you'll feel like dragging it out every time you want to use it, or will the process derail your workout efforts? Will that extra step work against you? And remember when you go old school and buy a treadmill—you've got a fixed amount of exercises and you're limited to them for the life of the machine. Get some exercise experience at a gym or group fitness classes and make your workouts a part of your lifestyle so that you know what you like before you buy.

IF IT LOOKS GOOD, YOU'LL FEEL GOOD GOING THERE

Like any other room in your house that you decorate, you want to create the right environment in your home gym. You can enhance your space with mirrors, a great sound system, a cheerful paint color, a DVD player, and a flat screen television. However you decorate, you want to make it a place you enjoy being in so when you spend time there you get a great workout. It should be designed to be motivating and inspiring. Don't let yourself get overstimulated in the room either—think Zen. Have space available for your heart monitor, towels, and bottled water as well. And if it looks and feels great, maybe you'll feel excited enough to have friends come

Top Features of Well-designed Equipment:

1. FLEXIBILITY with machine—How many different exercises can you do? Can you grow and vary your workout with this machine? How many exercises per body part? What can you add to it? How many variations of an exercise can you do?

2. EASY TO MOVE—Can you move the apparatus around the room if you need to?

3. USER WEIGHT—Consider all the members of your family who will use the equipment. Is the equipment small enough to start with for the smaller members of the family that require a lower weight? Will it also be good for the stronger family members?

4. SPACE NEEDED—Do you have enough room available in your home? Front-facing equipment can be placed up against the wall or can fit in the corner of a room versus equipment that requires space on all sides.

5. MEETS YOUR GOALS—Have a goal in mind when you go to the store to purchase the equipment. Have clarity—do you want to lose ten pounds or do you want to gain strength? Do you want both?

6. EXTRA EQUIPMENT to add—Adding pieces of equipment adds flexibility to your routine, which enables you to balance all of your muscles. It's important to balance the muscles of your chest, back, legs, and arms so your structure stays balanced. The more exercises that are available to you, the more muscles you will use and the more likely you are to achieve a balanced workout. That's the bonus of functional strength-training equipment—it grows with you and gives you endless options.

7. QUALITY—Spend that little bit extra to buy a strong, sturdy piece of equipment. If you buy the least expensive piece on the floor, you'll likely get a shorter life span out of it. You want something that will last at least ten years.

8. LOW MAINTENANCE—The treadmill takes the most work to clean because of the belt. Dust can get trapped and affect the movement, so you need to wipe it down every month or two. Make sure your gym is in a dry place as well, which will extend the life of the equipment. Keep your pieces covered so you don't have the kids and pets playing on them or dust piling up. Service your equipment once a year.

9. USER FRIENDLY—Make sure you buy equipment that you fully understand how to use. If you're not high-tech, don't buy a high-tech machine unless you are totally committed to understanding its use. Ask the salesperson for instructions—many pieces come with DVDs, and some come with wall charts to help accelerate your learning curve.

ESS Story: Theresa Houchin

The structure of my body was a mess. So I started with chiropractic care four years ago. I had hurt my back moving some furniture, and I was in horrible pain. I couldn't bend over, had a lot of pain sleeping, was unable to get my housework done, couldn't function at work, and couldn't partake in my favorite pastime, which is bowling. I was forty-five feeling, walking, and looking ninety-five years old.

My sister, who has been in the medical field for the past thirty years, told me that chiropractors couldn't fix what was wrong with my back and that I would have to go to a neurosurgeon and probably have back surgery. I resisted that temptation! Much to her disbelief, I started to feel better after just a few adjustments from my chiropractor Dr. Eric Becking in Jackson, Missouri, and also noticed other things with my health—that I didn't know chiropractic could help with—disappear. I had also been having other health issues like acid reflux, bronchitis every winter, sinus infections at least one time a year, leg cramps, earaches, and more than enough colds. I thought it was all a part of aging. Boy was I wrong. Throughout the past four years, since taking care of my structure, spine, and nerve system, I no longer have any of those symptoms.

I'm forty-eight, but I feel twenty-eight, and my children sometimes tell me I should act my age! I have been able to walk more, exercise more (we bought a Bowflex five years ago, and I enjoyed cleaning the dust off!), and have even bought exercise videos to keep moving and stay young. I have lost thirty-six pounds. I eat right, get plenty of exercise (I walk at least thirty minutes per day and work out on our Bowflex three to four times a week), get plenty of rest, and get adjusted on a regular basis. I can now work in my yard with my flowers, enjoy more physical activities, spend more time with my family, and not be so cranky because I didn't feel good. My attitude is a lot different than it was, as I feel healthier, laugh a lot, am more confident about myself, and can get around a lot better. I have gotten back the half inch of my height that I thought was gone. My bowling scores have even improved! I would not trade anything that I have done over the past four years and will continue all the elements of The 100 Year Lifestyle for the rest of my life.

over and work out with you. Create a space that will empower you to take your fitness to higher levels. Enhance the environment with a vision board, motivational sayings, or your goals. Keep changing them so that your environment stays fresh. Ask for fitness gifts to round out and complete your home gym.

DON'T FORGET ABOUT LOGISTICS

There are some technical things to keep in mind as well as aesthetic. You want proper flooring in your workout room. Rubber matting is easy to clean and won't get damaged if you drop a weight. Keep in mind that most cardio equipment has levelers to keep it stable and carpet makes it harder to level. You'll likely have to put a mat under any piece of equipment you buy. Another technical concern is the need for power. A treadmill, for example, requires a power source, so while the center of the basement sounds good, make sure you're near a plug. You also want to take noise into consideration. You can't set yourself up in a spare bedroom next to the kids' room if the equipment you've purchased is loud and you plan to work out after they are asleep.

Whatever you add or wherever you set up, make sure your home gym keeps your goals in mind and helps you live your ideal 100 Year Lifestyle. Make sure it's a place you feel passionate and excited about so using it is enjoyable for your body, mind, and spirit.

The downside to having a home gym is that you will need to be self-motivated. You can't beat the convenience, but you will probably work out alone more often than not. For some of you that's the exciting part. For others you may need the people contact and the stimulus that comes from belonging to a gym or attending a group fitness class. I believe the pros certainly outweigh the cons, and I also believe we will see the day when all newly built homes will have a space specifically designated for a home gym. Just like when sunrooms or home theaters dominated the new home market, I believe the next wave for the building industry will be going green and home gyms.

Maintain your gym membership if you have one and can afford to so that you can change your environment, learn about new equipment and fitness trends, and take some fitness classes. This may help you break through plateaus and vary your workouts to keep them fun and interesting.

UNLIMITED OPTIONS

The options for a home gym are almost unlimited. When you make fitness a part of your ideal 100 Year Lifestyle, you will realize that it is less about the equipment than it is about your commitment to the lifestyle. The equipment becomes the bonus. As the years go by and new technologies emerge, you will find yourself buying and selling equipment, trading up for newer models, and enjoying the entire experience.

The 100 Year Lifestyle is a fitness lifestyle. Bring it into your home and you will permanently eliminate any excuses, maximize your workouts, and get yourself in the best shape of your life.

CONCLUSION:

Be a Lifestyle Leader

Congratulations on completing this book. You are on your way. It is now time for you to become a lifestyle leader and spread the word. You can do this by talking to people about their longevity. Get them to see that they share the genes of their aging parents and grandparents and use this as leverage to get them to take action in the present and change their life.

As a lifestyle leader, you can bring this consciousness and The 100 Year Lifestyle to your company, school, associations, and your community. This is happening in communities around the globe. With health care reform on the horizon, we must all make the self-care reforms necessary to keep us healthy throughout our lifetime, and maximize our innate potential. Thank you for spreading the word.

Please visit www.100yearlifestyle.com on a regular basis to get updates on the latest menus, recipes, exercise and health tips, as well as the latest information on all of the elements of The 100 Year Lifestyle that will help you to live your best life, every day.

The 100 Year Lifestyle Workout will give you the endurance to live your extended life span with a strong kick at the finish line, the strength to be active and energetic, and the structure to stand strong regardless of your age. Challenge yourself by keeping your workouts fresh, trying new things, and testing the limits of your fitness capabilities. You will be amazed at how you can get stronger and healthier every year. Bring your family and friends along with you. It is my hope and prayer that you and your loved ones enjoy a sensational century.

See you there.

ACKNOWLEDGMENTS

This is my favorite section to write. I am filled with tremendous gratitude for all of the unconditional love, support, and confidence that my family, friends, and colleagues have shown me throughout the years.

My wife, Lisa, has been a rock for me and my family. She has always been a strong, honest, and loving voice that I can count on for truth. We have been married twenty-one years and are going strong, and I look forward to our sensational century together. My children, Jacob, Emily, and Cory, are my compass and constant source of inspiration and purpose. They have all embraced The 100 Year Lifestyle philosophy and are living fit and healthy lives. I continue to be proud of you not just because you are my children but because you are growing into fine young people with character. Continue to pursue your passions and enjoy your lifestyle.

To my mom, Barbara Plasker, thank you for your strength, your courage, and for passing on your passion for human potential. Thank you also for being there for me with your wisdom and for loving me unconditionally. Dad, I sure wish you could read this and I miss you more than you know. Your dementia has robbed the world of a kind, strong, compassionate man. I wish my children could have had more time with you. You are with me in my heart always and together it is my prayer that this work can save some lives. To my mother- and father-in-law, Joanne and Herb Singer, I enjoy our family dinners and appreciate the support you give our family. Here's to good health and many more good times together. To my brothers, Dr. Jordan Plasker and Dr. Noel Plasker, thank you for being my best friends.

To Jack LaLanne, your vision for longevity and human potential was way before its time. From your chiropractic college graduation to your decades of dedication to innovation in the fitness world, you have been a tremendous source of inspiration. To Roger Craig, thank you my friend for being a leader in professional sports by standing up for the chiropractic profession and working hard to make chiropractic care a core part of professional sports. I believe that your pioneering spirit is a main reason why DCs are working with professional, Olympic, college, high school, and youth sports teams worldwide.

To Dave Kenyon from Gold's Gym, thanks for your impeccable detail in organizing the photographs and being so passionate about The 100 Year Lifestyle. Thank you to photographer Alan Lemberger for taking great pictures and to our models who posed so beautifully for this book, Bill Young, Jessica Sledzianowski, Terri Sileno, Jeff Hartford, and Josh Johnson.

To the chiropractic profession and my chiropractic colleagues, I am grateful for our health and wellness principles and for the dedication that we all show to communities around the globe. We have been through many battles together and as the political landscape changes, may we continue to fight the good fights that stand for what is right in the world of health care while we maintain our core principles. There are so many chiropractors that I need to thank that I am sure I will leave some of you out, but let's give it a try. Thank you to Dr. Fabrizio Mancini, Parker College president, Dr. John Bueler, Dr. Dave Benevento, Dr. Maia James, Kim DeWeese, Scott Van Horn, and the entire board and membership of the California Chiropractic Association. Thank you to all the current members and executive committees of the ICA, ACA, WCA, WFC, ASRF, COCSA, ACC, and CCA, who have all supported The 100 Year Lifestyle on some level. That's a lot of initials.

To all my friends in the chiropractic media, thank you so much for helping to deliver this message around the world. To Jaclyn Busch Touzard and Dr. Joseph Busch of *The American Chiropractor,* your magazine is first class and I am honored to be one of your media consultants. To everyone at *Chiropractic Economics, The Chiropractic Journal, Dynamic Chiropractic, The Canadian Chiropractor,* and *Chiropractic Lifestyle* magazines, thanks for the opportunity to contribute and for trusting my voice.

Thank you to the College Presidents and grass roots leaders who run CORE, EPOC, and other chiropractic groups around the country including Dr. Matt Hubbard, Dr. Troy Dukowitz, Dr. Lyle Koca, Dr. Bill Demoss, Dr. Brad Glowaki, Dr. Ari Diskin, Dr. Gilles LaMarche, Dr. Larry Markson, Dr. Patrick Gentempo, Dr. Peter Kevorkian, Dr. Patti Giuliano, Dr. Jim Dubell, Dr. Mark Sanna, Dr. Tim Gay, Dr. Ernie Landi, Drs. Roy and Matt Sweat, Dr. Ciro Rustici, Dr. Guy Riekeman, president of Life University, Dr. Carl Cleveland, president of Cleveland Chiropractic College, Dr. Gerard Clum, president of Life Chiropractic College West and many others.

Thanks to the Foundation for Chiropractic Progress for their excellent public relations campaign which hopefully all doctors will continue to support.

Thank you to Dr. Carol Ann Malizia; I spelled your name right this time. I always appreciate your leadership, sisterly support, and friendship. Thanks to Doug Capporino for being a catalyst for my fitness journey.

Thank you also to the chiropractors who contributed content to *The 100 Year Lifestyle Workout* including Dr. Jeff Spencer, Dr. Pete Gratale, Drs. Terry and Lori Schroeder, Dr. Brian Jensen, and Dr. Tony Lauro of Stay Fit Seniors to name a few. Thank you also to the leaders of all of the chiropractic colleges and national and state associations. It is always a pleasure for me to speak to your students and alumni at conventions and in the classroom. I appreciate your open invitations.

Thank you to all of the individuals and companies who support The 100 Year Lifestyle including Kent Greenwald of Foot Levelers, Ron Rosenthal and Chuck Grossman from eyeQuest, Philip Mills of Les Mills, Mike Epstein, Bill Austin, Josh Wheeler, Dave Reisman, Todd Cioffi, Corry Matthews, and the rest of my friends at Gold's Gym. Thank you to Larry Domingo and Annie Beason from Precor, and Neal Spruce, Dr. Michael Clark, Ben Tucker, and Carol Schober from National Academy of Sports Medicine and dotFIT.

Thank you also to my book and public relations team including my agent, John Willig, Lara Asher and Scott Watrous from Globe Pequot, Robyn and Willy Spizman, Carly Felton, Stephanie Krikorian, Gary Krebs, as well as Paula Munier and the Adams Media team who continue to support and promote *The 100 Year Lifestyle*.

Thank you to all of the doctors who are becoming 100 Year Lifestyle Certified Providers and to our clients who continue to support this vision through their investment in our products and services. Thank you to my team at The Family Practice including Teri Bynum, Sergio Nascimento, Kimberly Brenowitz as well as our present and past coaches, Dr. Cheryl Langley, Dr. Miguel Cruz and Lesia Cruz, Dr. Russ Pavkov, Dr. Bart Rzepa, Drs. Scott and Betty Jo Clark, Dr. Glenn Lang, Dr. Gary Brodeur, Dr. Scott Stachelek, Dr. Carmello Caratozzolo, Dr. Terry Harmon, and Dr. Craig and Nicole Pruitt.

Thank you also to the many people who I have forgotten to mention who are important in my life.

INDEX

ABOUT THE AUTHOR

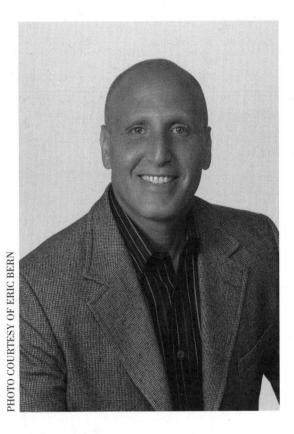

Eric Plasker, DC, inspires his patients and the public alike to realize "a long life, well-lived." A graduate of Life Chiropractic College and former owner of two highly successful family practices, Dr. Plasker is an internationally recognized speaker, media personality, and wellness expert. Featured on CNN, ABC, CBS, NBC, Fox, TBS, *Movie and a Makeover,* the Discovery Channel's *Forever Young* and Connecting with Kids television network, he's shared the stage with such luminaries as Dr. Wayne Dyer, Dr. Andrew Weil, and Dr. Barbara De Angelis to name a few. His health and wellness books, audio CDs, DVDs, and related materials have been translated into multiple languages and distributed in more than fourteen countries. Dr. Plasker's wellness messages reach millions of people around the world. He lives in Atlanta, Georgia. Visit www.100yearlifestyle.com to learn more.